T0100178

THE REAL
AIDS
EPIDEMIC

THE REAL AIDS EPIDEMIC

How the Tragic HIV Mistake Threatens Us All

Rebecca V. Culshaw

Foreword by Neenyah Ostrom

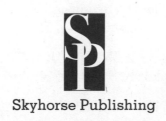

Skyhorse Publishing

Copyright © 2007, 2023 by Rebecca V. Culshaw
Foreword © 2023 by Neenyah Ostrom

All Rights Reserved. No part of this book may be reproduced in any manner without the express written consent of the publisher, except in the case of brief excerpts in critical reviews or articles. All inquiries should be addressed to Skyhorse Publishing, 307 West 36th Street, 11th Floor, New York, NY 10018.

Skyhorse Publishing books may be purchased in bulk at special discounts for sales promotion, corporate gifts, fund-raising, or educational purposes. Special editions can also be created to specifications. For details, contact the Special Sales Department, Skyhorse Publishing, 307 West 36th Street, 11th Floor, New York, NY 10018 or info@skyhorsepublishing.com.

Skyhorse® and Skyhorse Publishing® are registered trademarks of Skyhorse Publishing, Inc.®, a Delaware corporation.

Visit our website at www.skyhorsepublishing.com.

10 9 8 7 6 5 4 3 2 1

Library of Congress Cataloging-in-Publication Data
is available on file.

Hardcover ISBN: 978-1-5107-7671-5
eBook ISBN: 978-1-5107-7672-2

Printed in the United States of America

To my dad, Dr. Nicholas Gerard Culshaw—world adventurer, gentle warrior, champion of the scientific method. You taught me how to think and how to love. Memory Eternal.

I wish to acknowledge the invaluable assistance of the following people over the years, in alphabetical order: Elena A., Darin B., Henry B., Celia F., Matt I., Robert K., Sofia K., Kala M., Neenyah O., David R., Liam S., Nathan S., Val T., and, especially, Chuck.

Table of Contents

Foreword
by Neenyah Ostrom

Medical research, like most human endeavors, operates within a framework of conventional wisdoms. Partly because it impacts human lives directly—and partly because of the great wealth it can generate—medical research and its partner, medical practice, comply with their conventional wisdoms more strictly than other branches of science. Dissenting views and voices are not welcome.

Medicine's most rigidly adhered-to conventional wisdom of the last forty years is that the Human Immunodeficiency Virus, HIV, is the sole cause of AIDS.

Rebecca Culshaw is uniquely qualified to question that paradigm. With a PhD in Mathematical Biology, she upends the problematic arithmetic that supports the HIV hypothesis—the strangely unchanging number of HIV-positive people since the late 1980s, their location in the same geographical regions, occurring among the same "risk groups." She nullifies the certainty of the medical markers used to diagnose AIDS: the inexplicable loss of CD4+T cells, the fallacy of the viral load test, the weaknesses of PCR testing. In *The Real AIDS Epidemic*, Rebecca dismantles the conventional wisdom that rules HIV research.

Medical conventional wisdom is overturned only rarely, but we needn't revisit Galileo's seventeenth-century world to find examples: In the twentieth century, Australian researchers Professor Barry Marshall and Dr. Robin Warren were jeered when they produced evidence showing that ulcers are caused not by stress but by a bacterium, *Helicobacter pylori*. To prove their hypothesis, Professor Marshall swallowed three cultures of *H. pylori* in 1982, developed an ulcer, then biopsied and cultured the organism. In 2005, they were awarded the Nobel Prize in Medicine for their paradigm-busting discovery. And in the twenty-first century, the seemingly ironclad thesis that Alzheimer's disease is caused by plaques of amyloid protein is being questioned even in traditional journals like *Science*. Because anti-plaque medications destroyed them but patients' memories and cognitive abilities did not improve, the purported cause of Alzheimer's disease and the research surrounding it have come under serious scrutiny.

Before investigating the holes that riddle the HIV theory of AIDS, Rebecca was an assistant professor at the University of Texas at Tyler with a more than respectable list of publications. Her PhD research had involved constructing mathematical models of HIV infection. She was actively involved in peer review of mathematical and bio-mathematical research, having served on the editorial board of the *Journal of Biological Systems*. Upon publication of her essay, "Why I Quit HIV," the university began receiving coordinated warnings that she was a menace to society and a threat to the integrity of the university; she was falsely accused of giving medical advice to AIDS patients online. Her contract with the university was not renewed.

In *The Real AIDS Epidemic: How the Tragic HIV Mistake Threatens Us All,* Rebecca offers a blueprint for moving beyond the HIV paradigm. A first step would be a "Reproducibility Project" in AIDS research, focusing on the early papers from the National Cancer Institute laboratory of Robert Gallo, the "co-discoverer" of HIV, as well as influential—but often not reproduced—research reports from the mid-1990s.

Forty years after the press conference that announced HIV causes AIDS, the HIV theory has produced no vaccine and no cure, only the prospect of lifelong treatment with toxic anti-HIV medications. Many clinical trials of these noxious drugs are targeted at African American, gay, and impoverished individuals, including children born to HIV-positive mothers.

Instead of the promised cure, the 1980s brought patients monotherapy: the toxic and teratogenic AZT, with side effects of anemia, bone marrow suppression, and wasting symptoms. The 1990s brought multi-drug therapies called Highly Active AntiRetroviral Therapy (HAART), with side effects of kidney failure, loss of bone density and teeth, and disfiguring redistribution of body fat. Recently, two-drug combos like Dovato were developed, with side effects including anxiety, irregular heartbeat, liver disease, and more.

Today, anti-HIV therapies are directed toward currently healthy *HIV negative* individuals who are considered to be "at risk." Like the other anti-HIV therapies, Pre-Exposure Prophylaxis (PrEP) therapies are designed to be taken for life. And like the others, they are highly toxic. Most disturbingly, all advertising and public service announcements for PrEP target gay and African American populations—clearly reinforcing suspicions that the structure supporting the HIV paradigm is built on racism and homophobia.

In *The Real AIDS Epidemic*, you will read of lives destroyed by one of the PrEP drugs developed by pharmaceutical giant Gilead. Despite creating a "safer" version of its drug Truvada— "TAF"—Gilead declined to put it on the market until the patent on its first version of the drug, "TDF," expired. Developed in 2001, TDF causes serious side effects including osteoporosis leading to bone loss and tooth breakage, kidney disease leading to dialysis, and numerous interactions with other drugs. This marketing decision made in 2004 is the subject of a still-unsettled, more than 22,000-plaintiff class action lawsuit against Gilead.

A December 1, 2022 Reuters report revealed another profit motive most likely involved in Gilead's decision to run out TDF's patent before marketing TAF. The Centers for Disease Control and Prevention (CDC) is suing its collaborator Gilead for $1 billion in patent infringement for Truvada's use in PrEP. CDC contends Gilead did not credit the agency for discovering that Truvada could prevent HIV infection; Gilead alleges misconduct by CDC. A jury trial to determine which entity makes the most profit on PrEP is set for July 2023.

When in 1988 I began reporting on this rift in the medical community—between those who believed HIV alone causes all AIDS symptoms, allied against those who revealed data showing HIV to be peripheral if not unnecessary for AIDS to develop—I would not have believed it would stretch well into the next century. In 1995's *Censored: The News That Didn't Make The News And Why*, the *New York Native* and I were recognized for reporting the inaccuracy of HIV antibody tests. Almost thirty years later, HIV antibody tests are no more accurate. And, as was the case in 1995 and before, people who test negative for HIV antibodies can develop AIDS-like symptoms and impaired immune systems;

people who test positive for HIV antibodies can live long, healthy lives—if they don't take toxic anti-HIV drugs.

Along with those who worked beside me in New York City at the *New York Native* and elsewhere—John Lauritsen, Charles Ortleb, Celia Farber, Joan Shenton, Professors Peter Duesberg and Serge Lang, and a cadre of like-minded questioners across the globe—I was among the first generation of HIV whistleblowers.

Forty years later, Rebecca Culshaw is the vanguard of a second generation of HIV whistleblowers.

Will we need a third generation?

Neenyah Ostrom
Author of *America's Biggest Cover-Up: 50 More Things Everyone Should Know About the Chronic Fatigue Syndrome and Its Link to AIDS*; *Ampligen: The Battle for a Promising ME/CFS Drug*; and *Chronic Illness & HHV-6 Report* on SubStack.

Foreword to the Second Edition

When the first edition of this book, titled *Science Sold Out: Does HIV Really Cause AIDS?*, was published in 2007, I joined a long list of hopeful people who identified the many deadly flaws in the HIV=AIDS paradigm. We all hoped for a widespread and enthusiastic collective hearing of our whistleblowing, and that in the spirit of Thomas Kuhn, the paradigm would shift. Patients and the public would no longer be victims of fraud, incompetence, and deceit.

Clearly, time has taught us that we were far too optimistic. Things have dramatically worsened, and the shortfalls and corruption of government and pharmaceutical company–funded "science" have become obvious to many. It would be easy to brush my hands off and leave it to the next generation of doctors, scientists, and mathematicians to find and to fix what is broken.

But I can't sit idly by. Here we go again.

Author's Note

The real purpose of the scientific method is to make sure Nature hasn't misled you into thinking something you don't actually know. . . . If you get careless or go romanticizing scientific information, giving it a flourish here and there, Nature will soon make a complete fool of you. It does it often enough anyway even when you don't give it opportunities. One must be extremely careful and rigidly logical when dealing with Nature: one logical slip and an entire scientific edifice comes tumbling down. One false assumption about the machine and you can get hung up indefinitely.

—Robert Pirsig, *Zen and the Art of Motorcycle Maintenance*

Science is something more (and less) than the dispassionate pursuit of knowledge. How scientific information is shaped is often predetermined by the prevailing ideological climate. For centuries scientists have paid dearly for maintaining iconoclastic views. Their oppressors often have been other scientists working in tandem with the established powers in science.

—Michael Parenti, *Dirty Truths*

The purpose of this note is to explain a little about the format of this book, and certain logical assumptions that must be made.

I have in the past been accused of "trying to have it both ways," in particular concerning the issue of HIV's isolation. The argument has been made that I argue that HIV has not been proven to be isolated, yet at times I assume its existence when I point out anomalies in HIV/AIDS theory. As a mathematician, I know that one of the most powerful tools at our disposal is something called "proof by contradiction," and it involves assuming a certain fact to be true, then deriving a contradiction using the available evidence. If the information is self-falsifying, it therefore cannot be true. This is, in a nutshell, my approach to the HIV question. I don't have to prove it exists, or doesn't exist, but there is nothing inherently self-contradictory in assuming its existence in order to demonstrate that, if it does exist as a unique exogenous retrovirus, it cannot possibly accomplish what it is said to accomplish in terms of immune destruction. My primary goal, and in a way the only important goal I have, is to exonerate HIV of any culpability in causing any disease. There is nothing inherently illogical in this approach, and it has been standard in mathematical reasoning from time immemorial.

The other issue I would like to address right out of the gate is the elephant in the room that is COVID. I have been cautioned that if I am at all skeptical of COVID, I will be painted as a conspiracy theorist. I want to make one thing crystal clear right now, and that I am in no way saying or implying that COVID doesn't exist or that there was no pandemic. On the contrary, I believe that something unusual was indeed happening in early 2020 and most likely had begun in the fall of 2019. My primary concern with COVID "science" was the fact that the PCR test was being used to quantify the epidemic in a way that was at best inaccurate and at worst dishonest. Further to that, mathematical models were widely misused and abused to make continually failing predictions in a way that was transparently fraudulent, and had the net effect of making people more, not less, suspicious of the utility of mathematical modeling. Finally, and this is critical because it absolutely parallels AIDS and the fast-tracked approval of AZT in the 1980s, HAART in the 1990s, and PrEP/PEP today, is the fact that in rushing to approve mRNA vaccines for COVID, what was essentially a massively unethical clinical trial was conducted in real time on the entire population. The dangers of the vaccines are well known now, particularly among younger populations, but recall how quickly the "science" changed regarding COVID.

This is not the first time that this has happened. It is just the first time people began to realize that not being in a "risk group" didn't make them immune to being used as pawns in a very high stakes game.

Lastly, the blatant vilification and censorship of *scientists* who did not follow lockstep with the mainstream COVID narrative—including Dr. Robert Malone, who was involved in the invention of the mRNA technology and dared to be skeptical of its use—is terribly familiar to those of us that endured similar vilification regarding our views on HIV. Science does not take place in a vacuum where we must not dare to disagree even on details, let alone the big picture. What began with AIDS continues to this day. We have a rare moment of opportunity, in which many people have woken up to the "science by consensus" that has infected so many government agencies and even some universities. The mismanagement of COVID is the reason people are awake. Let's not fall back to sleep.

The Racist and Homophobic Underpinnings of HIV/AIDS Theory

HIV didn't suddenly pop out of the rain forest or Haiti. It just popped into Bob Gallo's hands at a time when he needed a new career. It has been here all along. Once you stop looking for it only on the streets of the big cities, you notice that it is thinly distributed everywhere.

—Kary Mullis, *Dancing Naked in the Mind Field*

We are now forty years into AIDS. Many people reading this volume have never known a life without AIDS. Given the many, many billions of dollars spent on AIDS research and AIDS activism, which settled into one narrow channel of investigation regarding disease mechanism and causation—the narrow focus on the loss of CD4+ T cells and the hunt for an agent that might be attracted to them, effectively brushing aside any other immunological disruptions in favor of the T-cell depletion model—it is reasonable to ask what we have accomplished in forty years.

Forty years later, prevalence of HIV-positivity has remained identical at about one million Americans, utterly perplexing for a virus that is meant to be contagious, but does not behave that way epidemiologically. Furthermore, we have no vaccine although one was promised to be available in the 1980s. We have no cure, only treatments that are toxic and meant to be lifelong. The lack of a vaccine has not stopped the public health experts and the pharmaceutical industry from simply prescribing AIDS *treatments* as AIDS *preventatives*. The aggressive marketing of these so-called AIDS preventatives to marginalized communities should raise alarm and suspicion in anyone with even a cursory knowledge of recent medical history.

The HIV theory of AIDS has been constructed entirely around a groundless base of racism and homophobia. I don't say this lightly.

Most Americans—and indeed, most people—are well familiar with the Tuskegee syphilis experiment. This study was pioneered in 1932 and continued until 1972 with the stated intention of "studying the natural history of syphilis specifically, how syphilis evolves when untreated." The study was a joint effort between the United States Public Health Service, the Centers for Disease Control and Prevention, and Tuskegee University, a Black college in Alabama. There were six hundred total participants, selected specifically from the African American community. Three hundred and ninety-nine subjects had syphilis. Participants in this study who had syphilis were followed without being told the true nature of the study and were excluded from treatment without their knowledge. The Public Health Service deceived them as to the nature of the study. They were denied informed consent, and, more grievously, were not offered treatment with penicillin, which was known by 1947 to be an effective treatment for syphilis. Over one hundred men enrolled in this study died of syphilis as a result. This study is widely considered to be one of the most egregious breaches of medical ethics in recent history. In 1997, President Bill Clinton issued a formal apology to those victimized by this study.[1]

The study does not, unfortunately, represent an isolated incident but remains only one among many studies undertaken without much consideration for ethical research.

In the 1940s, US researchers intentionally infected Guatemalans from underserved communities such as prisons and mental health facilities with STDs. Sex workers were infected with gonorrhea and syphilis, and the participants in the study were then exposed to these sex workers. Again, no informed consent was given.[2]

More recently, in 2003, the late investigative reporter Liam Scheff broke a story about orphans in New York City taking part in AIDS drug trials without proper ethical standards and ending with great harm. In case we might wonder whether Tuskegee or the Guatemala study were simply products of their time, the story of the Incarnation Children's Center (ICC) serves as a reminder that public health officials are still conducting medical research in an unethical way among marginalized people.[3]

Children at the ICC were typically born to HIV-positive mothers and removed from their homes by Child Protective Services. They were typically Black or Hispanic and poor. While at the ICC, children became subjects in drug trials sponsored by none other than the National Institute of Allergies and Infectious Disease (NIAID). The drugs came with severe side effects, and compliance was low for this reason. (This will become a theme in AIDS drug trials.) Never to be stopped, however; if a child refused their medication, they were held down and force fed. If, under these circumstances they continued to refuse their medication, they had a tube surgically inserted into their intestines so that noncompliance would, at long last, not be an issue. Several children died—not of AIDS itself but of strokes due to the toxic nature of these drugs.

As just one example, Scheff interviewed the adoptive mother of two of these orphans. One of the children had been on AZT monotherapy from five months of age, and had twice been on life support as a direct result of the AIDS drug nevirapine, which gained notoriety following Celia Farber's coverage of the pregnant Joyce Ann Hafford in 2006. The other child has developed cancer despite being asymptomatic with respect to their HIV status at the time of treatment initiation.

The BBC eventually picked the story up and ran it as a documentary, "Guinea Pig Kids," but it was too late for those children who became ill and died as a direct result of the "lifesaving" HIV drugs.

Indeed, AIDS drug trials seem to have a common theme of a treatment being touted as the next best thing, only to discover— too late!—that they have side effects that are arguably worse than "living with HIV" which itself ceased being the same disease we saw in the 1980s, as long-term survivors of ten to twenty years or more became quite obvious by the mid-1990s—before the advent of highly active antiretroviral therapy (HAART) in 1996. (AIDS deaths actually peaked in 1993–94 and have dropped ever since. This is largely due to the CDC redefinition and extensive *widening* of the criteria for an AIDS diagnosis and is examined in more detail in chapter 4 of the main text.) We saw this with AZT monotherapy in the early nineties, for example, and we continue to see this.

Fast forward to 2021. Tyreese Buchanan, a San Diego man who was diagnosed HIV-positive in 2001, went public as the face of a 21,000-person class action lawsuit against the drug manufacturer Gilead because of the debilitating side effects he and other patients have experienced as a result of the anti-HIV drugs Truvada and Viread (TDF). Buchanan used to be a singer who loved to perform, but he rarely leaves his home anymore. He has experienced kidney failure and bone density and tooth loss. "It hurts your pride . . . [it's] like someone stabbed me with a butcher knife in the hip."[4]

He is hardly close to being the only victim, as this class action lawsuit engages 22,000 plaintiffs. Legal counsel for the plaintiffs maintain that Gilead gave the study participants a less safe version of the AIDS drug tenofovir, called TDF, for years to maximize profits despite the fact that they were knowingly withholding an allegedly safer version of tenofovir, known as TAF. Gilead insisted on providing tenofovir until its patent expired, despite TAF being available and allegedly safer.

The 22,000 plaintiffs in this lawsuit have suffered severe bone loss and kidney damage due to the toxicity of TDF. People have broken bones walking up stairs, and have lost teeth simply from biting a piece of fruit. The lawsuit is ongoing.

It is worth asking the question of whether TAF is truly a safe alternative. Most of these drugs were optimistically presumed to be safe in their early days, but time does seem to have a way of disproving such claims.

As well, it is notable that TDF is widely prescribed as part of Pre-Exposure Prophylaxis (PrEP) even today, despite ongoing allegations of serious adverse events. PrEP is not to be confused with

Post-Exposure Prophylaxis (PEP), which is like a morning after pill for patients who had reason to believe they had been exposed to HIV, and is only prescribed transiently. PrEP, on the other hand, is specifically targeted toward healthy, HIV-negative individuals believed to be "at risk" for acquisition of HIV positivity.

I don't think that it can be overstated how bizarre and unprecedented it is in medical history to put healthy individuals *on toxic chemotherapy for life*. The closest parallel I can imagine is the widespread use of hormonal contraceptives among women, which is acknowledged by the World Health Organization to be a Class A carcinogen and is falling out of favor among women. We will examine the medical and statistical underpinnings of PrEP in the section "Fake Science."

Meanwhile, television and print advertisements for HAART and PrEP are problematic. They feature pleasant looking, active people—most of whom are African American—living their best lives on a daily regime of so-called anti-HIV drugs, while the voice-over tells quite a different story. "PrEP may not be for everyone," "PrEP has not been shown to be effective among transgender women," and so forth, followed by the standard laundry list of side effects recited at a rapid pace due to the sheer number of them. In my opinion, these advertisements are no better than promotion of the Tuskegee syphilis experiment. They are deceptive, and sneakily target the African American population.

We are told that AIDS drugs are safe. It is a lie. We are told that AIDS drugs save lives, although the only clinical endpoint taken into consideration is "viral load," with the holy grail of HIV treatment being "getting to undetectable [viral load value]." But the so-called HIV viral load test itself is of highly dubious quality, producing false positive results even in HIV-negative individuals.[5] The use of viral load as a clinical endpoint itself is rather bizarre, as it only became widely used in 1996, which was *after* life expectancies of HIV-positive individuals had dramatically increased from the one- to three-year estimate at the beginning of the AIDS epidemic to ten to fifteen years or more. Again, HAART only came into prominence in 1997, while AIDS deaths had begun to decline in the mid 1990s. Given the long latent period of "HIV disease," this cannot possibly be due to drug treatment, since these people had supposedly been HIV-positive since at least the mid 1980s if not earlier.

In this introduction, I hope to make the following points crystal clear:

The HIV causes AIDS paradigm is at its heart racist and antigay. I believe that, for complicated sociological reasons, large subsections of these populations are experiencing a kind of Stockholm Syndrome at the hands of the scientific and medical communities. Using gay and African American people as guinea pigs continues, unfortunately, to this day.

We tend to believe that we are more ethical and more sensitive to the plight of minority and underserved populations than we were when the Tuskegee experiment evolved, but in reality, little has changed.

The African American community disproportionately tests positive for antibody to HIV across every risk group and geographical location in a way quite unlike infectious diseases including STIs, suggesting that elevated levels of HIV antibody may simply be more common in this population for some as yet unknown genetic reason.[6]

I contend that HIV testing and the use of AIDS drugs, especially the push for widespread use of PrEP, is a colossal and dangerous scam. We might have, at one time, thought such a scam to be an isolated incident that happens only to certain unlucky risk groups. To that I would caution that no one is without risk of being victimized by public health interventions that later turn out to be harmful.

One doesn't have to look back far into our collective history to recall that in late 2020 and into 2021, governments of countries around the world, in conjunction with various pharmaceutical companies, launched what was effectively a worldwide, billion-person clinical trial in real time, when the "lifesaving COVID vaccines" (note the language) were rolled out despite extremely limited testing. Regardless of one's position on either COVID or vaccines, there is little doubt that these "vaccines" (many of which are not vaccines in the traditional sense) emphatically do not do what they were advertised to do. The goalposts continue to be moved—from preventing infection, to preventing hospitalization, to preventing "long COVID"—and real accounts continue to mount of real, previously healthy and mostly young people suffering severe side effects as a result of these injections.

The push for widespread PrEP uptake is reminiscent of the COVID vaccine controversy. Focus is moving away from real clinical endpoints entirely in favor of widespread prescription of so-called anti-HIV medications, despite the side effects that we see clearly, and despite the patent ridiculousness of putting perfectly healthy people on chemotherapy *for life.*

The AIDS crisis has been used to ghettoize and victimize gay and African American people. The COVID crisis has proven that this can happen to anyone. No one is immune to governmental and medical coercion.

We've Seen This Before

Attacks on me are, quite frankly, attacks on science.
—Anthony Fauci, December 2021

In March of 2020, public health officials cautioned the world that "social distancing" would remain our best defense against COVID19, until such time as the miracle vaccines would arrive. People stayed home; schools, businesses, and places of worship were closed; elderly and critically ill people were denied the company of their loved ones in order to "keep them safe," only for many of them to die, tragically, alone; and, ridiculously, we were advised to maintain a distance of six feet apart—for an airborne pathogen. Countries like Australia, the UK, and Canada issued exorbitant fines to anyone caught disobeying the rules. People were quarantined, actually locked inside quarantine facilities, simply for testing positive on a PCR test (which is the identical technology used to estimate "viral load"). Of course, we now know that many of these public health officials and politicians were not actually following their own guidelines. As just one example, the former prime minister of the UK, Boris Johnson, himself resigned in disgrace amid the "PartyGate" scandal.

The "six feet" figure was obviously made up, especially considering it is well known that respiratory viruses are airborne and circulate especially well indoors, where six feet or ten feet are probably about the same. People, breathing through cloth masks or at best, ill-fitting N95s, dutifully protected one another by standing six feet apart. We end up with footprints on the floors of stores that remain in place today.

Then, in late 2020, the long-awaited (for nine whole months) COVID vaccinations were rolled out. Surely part of the reason for the eager initial uptake of these injections was the desperate desire to return to a sense of normalcy after months of social isolation. How popular would these shots have been were it not for the natural desire to simply live a normal life?

Regardless of the reason, initial uptake of these shots was impressive. Originally touted as "safe and effective," we were told at first that if we got vaccinated, we would not contract COVID. This was quickly proven to be false, as quite rapidly, vaccinated or unvaccinated, almost everyone got COVID. The narrative was then switched and we were told that the vaccinations would prevent "severe illness." When this too was shown to be false, and following numerous reports of severe adverse events and death, we were told that the vaccines represented the best protection against "long COVID" (another ill-defined syndrome not dissimilar to AIDS). Here we are nearly two years later, and only 3 percent of the population is taking advantage of the so-called "booster" shots. This is true even in states such as California and Massachusetts, where people were generally happier to "follow the science" than those in more rural or right-leaning states.

We have had two years of vaccine mandates, and to what end? Are we better off? Perhaps in a way we are, as large portions of the population have come to realize that the politicians, public health officials, and drug manufacturers essentially ran a 1 billion plus person, global clinical trial that failed in real time. Further, in early October 2022, an executive for Pfizer pharmaceuticals admitted that their clinical trials had *never tested the vaccines' efficacy regarding transmission.* The observant reader might point out in actuality, "the science" never addressed this, and this is the excuse now being given to address the shots' lack of efficacy. "The science didn't actually say that." No, it did not, but that did not stop public health officials from stating on television that when one gets vaccinated, they are a "dead end to the virus."

We see a pattern here. Something is announced and put into place based on flimsy evidence and wishful thinking. Any question on these issues comes with a resounding condemnation—how dare anyone question the domain experts? Science denier! The scientists and experts who criticize publicly are villainized and told to "stay in their lanes." Thus a house is constructed on sand, whether "six feet seems about right," or running a massive clinical trial on the global population based only on the results of small underpowered studies that should not be extrapolated to different populations on different continents. Yet, years later, the footprints remain on the floor.

Throughout the COVID pandemic, and especially at the beginning, the use of mathematical (computer) models was extremely popular as a method for predicting the course of the pandemic and for estimating the efficacies of particular interventions. Many of these models turned out to be comically wrong, but their misuse continues.

The real issue with models is not that they can be inaccurate—which is certainly the case—but that, *by their very design*, they can only produce results that depend on the information used to construct the models. More precisely, they only spit out what is put in (hence the term "garbage in, garbage out"). Their true utility is in estimating the magnitude of the effect that certain interventions, abstracted as parameters or functions, have on the system being modeled. They cannot tell you *whether* a particular intervention will work; they can only assume that it will and provide an estimate as to how much of an effect they will have. A model that predicts that social distancing or vaccines will work *necessarily* assumes at the outset, *as a condition of the model*, that the intervention will have a certain effect. This concept is especially important when it comes to HAART and, most especially, to PrEP.

Many people the world over have grown more and more horrified that they were duped into taking a vaccine that doesn't work and can in some cases cause great harm, on the basis of a lie. Imagine how much worse it will be when hundreds of thousands to millions of people were administered *toxic chemotherapy on a daily basis for life*, to prevent the acquisition of a status—HIV-antibody-positivity—for which there is no evidence that it can be prevented pharmaceutically. (Indeed, efficacy of condoms is generally considered to be higher, at 90 percent, than that of PrEP.)

Fake Science

We know that to err is human, but the HIV/AIDS hypothesis is one hell of a mistake.
    —Kary Mullis, foreword to *Inventing the AIDS Virus*
                                            by Peter Duesberg

We are being fed a diet of "fake science." COVID has been the event that was so blatant and in your face that many people have come to realize that "trust the experts" isn't necessarily the best advice, for many reasons, but in particular because data are tremendously easy to manipulate, particularly as one moves out of the realm of reality and into that of abstraction. The HIV theory of AIDS has been extremely abstract from the beginning. However, there remain three indisputable facts about the HIV theory of AIDS that remain true forty years into the epidemic.

- As the late Kary Mullis—inventor of the PCR test that has been the foundation of both AIDS and COVID treatment and diagnosis—pointed out thirty years ago, there is no paper nor *collection of papers, taken together* that establishes what we have been conditioned to believe: that HIV is the probable cause of AIDS.

- There remains no plausible mechanism of action for the T-cell depletion seen in AIDS. HIV has never been shown to destroy T-cells in culture, and there is no consensus or even a unified theory of how HIV mediates this destruction. Like so many other aspects of HIV theory, it is simply assumed to be true.

- Bizarrely, in the popular literature we see less and less emphasis on T-cell depletion as one of the sequelae of alleged HIV infection, in favor of the theory that HIV actually causes *massive inflammation,* leading to cancer and cardiovascular ailments. This is truly perplexing for several reasons—first, inflammation tends to be indicative of an *over*active immune system, not one that has been entirely decimated as we have been told is the hallmark of AIDS. Second, and this is crucially important—the *entire reason* HIV was even considered as a potential cause for AIDS is that the observation of CD4+ T cell depletion led researchers to look for a pathogen that was attracted to these cells. Had they been looking for an agent that caused massive inflammation, would HIV have even made the short list?

- There is still no animal model for AIDS. HIV introduced into macaques, the closest feasible relative of humans for the purposes of experimentation, has never managed to cause AIDS in these animals.

Without repeating entire parts of the body of this volume, I would like to briefly summarize the primary scientific sources for the various AIDS treatments and interventions and present evidence that the primary sources in the scientific literature do not justify the treatments that they claim to support.

The first such papers were the infamous Gallo et. al. *Science* papers that were published in 1984 *after* the cause of AIDS had been announced via press conference. Putting aside the oddity of announcing the cause of a devastating disease to the entire world in advance of any supporting evidence being published in the literature, I will point out only that in his seminal paper that is most frequently cited as the answer to bullet point number one, he only found any trace of HIV in twenty-six out of seventy-two AIDS patients.[7]

This is the paper that launched this entire mess, and it is on the basis of this paper and its siblings that the HIV antibody test was developed. I won't go into the numerous issues with the HIV antibody tests (refer to chapter 5 in the main text) but will only mention one: that blood samples drawn for an initial HIV antibody test must be diluted by a factor of *four hundred*. This is significantly higher than dilution factors for any other diagnostic test, most of which do not require dilution at all. The reason it must be diluted so much is that, undiluted, *everyone will test positive for HIV.*[8] Nevertheless, this test is still in use today, despite the strong evidence the dilution factor yields that this test is most likely detecting elevated levels of non-specific antibodies.

The Gallo papers and those that built on their results were also the basis for the prescription of AZT monotherapy in the early days of the epidemic. AZT monotherapy is never used anymore due to its toxicity, and when AZT is given as part of a drug cocktail, it is at doses far lower than initially given.

The current treatment of choice for HIV remains highly active antiretroviral therapy, or HAART, which involves prescription of cocktails of anti-HIV drugs from the moment one tests positive. Given the latency period of AIDS, and the fact that it appears to be ever-lengthening, and was in fact lengthening already years prior to the advent of HAART, one can only surmise how profitable treatment with multiple chemotherapeutic drugs for *decades* would be for the companies producing such therapies.

What is often not mentioned to the general public is that the entire justification for HAART comes from two papers published in 1996 that have been widely debunked.[9,10] These were the papers of Ho and Wei published in *Nature*, which popularized the use of the "viral load" test and "hit hard, hit early" combination therapy. Viral load, despite being completely inappropriate to use to quantify anything *due to the very nature of the test*, is now *the* clinical endpoint used to make all treatment decisions for the patient.

Again, as Kary Mullis, the inventor of PCR (which is the basis of the viral load test), has stated, "quantitative PCR is an oxymoron." This is because, as many are now familiar due to the unreliability of the PCR test for COVID diagnosis, PCR amplifies genetic material by factors of 35–45, meaning that whatever genetic material was present initially, the final result of the PCR test will produce 235 to 245 to times the amount of genetic material that is actually there, which by its very nature will amplify any errors in counting by that magnitude. Common estimates for the HIV viral load test is that it overstates the actual amount of genetic material by a factor of 60,000. So a "viral load" of 60,000 corresponds to one infectious viral particle.

Nevertheless, the desired clinical endpoint in HIV treatment involves "getting to undetectable [viral load]"—when in fact a viral load of 60,000 is for all intents and purposes, undetectable. The *entire point* of using PCR for viral load measurements is that without PCR, most people will in fact be undetectable!

Furthermore, it has been shown that HIV-negative people *frequently* measure positive viral load values, which is why viral load is never used to diagnose HIV infection. In the 1998 paper by Mendoza et. al. [5], twenty HIV-antibody-negative low risk individuals were tested for viral load using three different commercial tests. On the first test, two of twenty people showed positive viral loads of 10,620 and 2,020. On the second, again two patients tested positive with viral load values of 150 and 480. Finally, on the last test, four people tested positive.

We also note that the entire mathematical basis behind HAART was given in the form of a model presented in the paper by Ho and Shaw in *Nature*, which is bankrupt.

> I have completed a preliminary analysis of the papers by Ho and Shaw which appeared in *Nature*, January 12, 1995. My considered opinion is that they are total rubbish. I seriously doubt that the two groups really have any idea what they are doing when they construct their supposed models of the interaction of the virus and the immune system. The models when analyzed properly do not do what they think they do.
>
> —Mark Craddock, 1995

Mark Craddock, the Australian mathematician quoted above, provides an excellent critique of this model, which I shall summarize by saying only that, given the assumptions of their model, AIDS should develop within *at most* sixty days of infection—AIDS in this case being defined as the *complete loss of every T-cell in the body*.

No wonder they promoted the "hit hard, hit early" treatment approach!

Given this information, the use of these tests in making clinical decisions would appear to be highly suspect and the argument could be made that these tests qualify legally as defective products that would be excellent candidates for a class action lawsuit (similar to the Gilead lawsuit) on behalf of patients whose treatment is managed largely or even exclusively on the results of this test, which should from the start have been determined unfit for its intended use. Please refer to chapter five of the main text for more in depth analysis of the viral load tests.

The next frontier in "HIV prevention," approved in 2012, is the medication of *healthy, HIV-negative* people with anti-HIV drugs in order to prevent the acquisition of HIV among members of risk groups. Setting aside the concern regarding putting healthy people on chemotherapeutic drugs for life and the attendant enormous profits for the drug manufacturers, the question is: Does this intervention even work?

I would like to draw attention once again to the Gilead lawsuit—22,000 individuals on Truvada, the drug of choice for pre-exposure prophylaxis (PrEP), all of whom were injured by Truvada, some in debilitating ways. We are told that there is a safer alternative, but given how HIV treatment changes constantly and the justification behind it remains ephemeral, it would not be out of line to wonder how safe, really, are the new treatments? They are not radically different biochemically from earlier iterations of these drugs, so to assume a level of safety far above any that has been demonstrated so far would appear to be nothing more than wishful thinking.

The elephant in the room that must be addressed is the picture we have been given of these drugs always being safe and effective, when all the while public health authorities are basically conducting a massive clinical trial in real time. The successive failures of the "lifesaving" COVID vaccines to meet their ever-evolving clinical endpoints should serve as a cautionary tale. We really *don't* know how safe and effective these medications are in the long term. We are finding this out as we go along.

Regardless, it is instructive to examine the results of several clinical trials that are commonly used to justify the use of PrEP by citing high efficacy at preventing HIV transmission, to see how high this efficacy really is.

I will make one point before (briefly) diving into some numbers. For this next section, it is imperative that I assume that there is a phenomenon of HIV-positivity that may be transmissible *even though this may not be true.* This does not make it true that HIV-positivity is transmissible; it simply *assumes* that it is, and then, using that assumption, purports to show that the medications under consideration are not as effective as claimed. This initial assumption is necessary as we attempt to debunk a paradigm "from the inside."

One curiosity encountered can be found in noting that the biggest decreases in HIV incidence among risk groups is in intravenous drug users, despite there being no evidence in the medical literature of PrEP's effectiveness in that particular risk group.

Let's dive into the results of some of the more well-respected clinical trials used to promote PrEP among men who have sex with men, transgender women, and heterosexual couples in Africa. In particular, we will examine the claim that PrEP is "99 percent effective" in preventing acquisition of HIV-positivity.

Given the actual results of these clinical trials, not to mention the level of attrition, which in itself suggests the side effects to be significant, and keeping in mind other similar results in recent medical history, it seems that a large dose of skepticism and caution is warranted.

A monograph published by AIDS United and ACT NOW: END AIDS and sponsored by the Ryan White Foundation called "Ending the HIV Epidemic in the United States: A Roadmap for Federal Action" strongly promotes PrEP as the key to ending HIV by either 2025 or 2035. A look at this document is illuminating, and the section titled "Modeling Public Health Goals for Ending the United States HIV Epidemic" caught my eye.[11]

In "Pillar 1: commit to end the US HIV epidemic and eliminate HIV health disparities," the stated goals are to "achieve the 95-95-95 care framework and 40 percent PrEP coverage by 2025." The so-called 95-95-95 care framework consists of having 95 percent of all HIV-antibody-positives knowing their status, 95 percent of those patients being "retained in care" (but "care" consists merely of compliance to HAART), and 95 percent of those "retained in care" achieving "viral suppression," which is commonly considered having a "viral load" of less than 20 copies per milliliter.

Current estimates consider that about one in eight HIV-antibody-positive individuals in the US are unaware of their status, implying that 87.5 percent of people *are* aware of their status. Of these, only 50 percent were retained in care, and 56 percent of those retained in care were virally suppressed.

If these drugs are so wonderful, why are only half of all HIV-positives who know their status taking them? The rate of "viral suppression" falls woefully short of the 95 percent ideal, as well, at barely more than half.

When it comes to PrEP, the uptake is even more dismal. According to a press release from Gilead Pharmaceuticals, "State of the HIV Epidemic,"[12] it is stated that 1.1 million Americans are eligible for PrEP based on risk factors, but in 2016, only 78,360, or less than 8 percent, even filled prescriptions. That estimate has increased to a rate of prescriptions issued (note that this is not the same as prescriptions *filled*) of about 25 percent.

Clinical trials that estimate the efficacy of PrEP have significant variability in the results. In the IPrEx study,[13] for men who have sex with men, a range of efficacies was given based on estimated adherence. Adherence was measured in three ways—self-report, pill count, and blood detection of the drug, and efficacies in these categories ranged from 50 percent to 92 percent, although the conclusion of this study was apparently derived by *inferring* that, if the drug were taken daily, efficacy would be 99 percent, despite 99 percent having been achieved nowhere in the study. It should be noted as well that the iPrEx study used the "older," less safe, version of tenofovir, TDF. Despite TAF being allegedly "safer," TDF remains widely prescribed.

A follow-up to the iPrEx study, in 2015,[14] enrolled 339 transgender women in a trial to evaluate the effectiveness of PrEP, and *no protective benefit was identified*. It was speculated that this was due to lower adherence.

Among heterosexual men and women,[15] efficacy of PrEP was estimated at about 75 percent, in the Partners PrEP study. In the TDF2 study, efficacy was found to be between 62 and 78 percent.

Among injection drug users in Bangkok,[16] PrEP effectiveness was estimated to be about 49 percent, which is significantly lower than among MSM or heterosexuals. This is interesting in and of itself because since the advent of PrEP, the risk group experiencing the largest decline in HIV-positivity was intravenous drug users, despite PrEP not being terribly effective in that population.

It appears clear that any miraculous benefits of PrEP are mostly in the minds of the drug manufacturers and researchers with a vested interest in this treatment modality. And we are nowhere near the

40 percent PrEP coverage envisioned in the Vivent Health/Ryan White document. This is certainly not due to lack of awareness, as advertisements for PrEP shamelessly target the African American community. This is perhaps a miscalculation, as African Americans are well aware of how they have been historically mistreated by the medical community, and understandably have a much higher level of suspicion. The ongoing Gilead lawsuit targeting the use of TDF serves as a cautionary tale. TAF may appear safer, but how many times has a new treatment come along that is touted as safe and effective, only to fall out of favor due to its toxicity profile and/or lack of effectiveness?

The push for widespread PrEP coverage continues, and is becoming more and more aggressive, with "compliance" the ultimate goal. To that end, "long lasting, injectable PrEP" is being marketed under brand names such as Apretude, a bimonthly injection given indefinitely. Furthermore, there is a push to link one's PrEP use to a phone app, so that compliance can be tracked. Interestingly, in trials comparing Apretude to Truvada, Apretude users had *higher* levels of adverse effects than did Truvada (TDF) users, which is alarming considering the safety profile of Truvada is not stellar.

Returning to the Ryan White document, we find several graphs of HIV prevalence and incidence over time, with nice colored lines representing what this curve will look like if we continue current standard of care versus achieving the 95-95-95 framework by 2025 and 2030 respectively. Another graph representing "bending the curve [sound familiar?] with PrEP" shows an astonishing drop in new infections that appears to be no more than wishful thinking, as evidenced by the fact that most people eligible for PrEP appear not to be too interested in taking it. One can speculate as to the reasons why, but it is perhaps the case that historically marginalized and mistreated communities might be suspicious of a regime that tracks their adherence to lifelong chemotherapy with well documented toxicities, especially if they are not even sick or HIV-positive to begin with. If the targeted communities knew how untrustworthy the science was, many more would be unwilling to participate in this potentially tragic experiment.

AIDS Has Changed

If you treat only healthy people you can claim great therapeutic success.

—Claus Kohnlein, 2005

This topic is covered extensively in chapter four of the original text, so I will discuss it only briefly here. It is my contention that AIDS in the early 1980s is not the same disease or even the same syndrome as it is now, or even as it was by the early 1990s. In the early 1980s, the latency period between infection and full-blown AIDS was estimated to be between one and three years, and the diseases that proved fatal were pneumocystis pneumonia, candidiasis, and Kaposi's sarcoma, the latter of which is rarely seen anymore and is not even attributed to HIV any longer. Globally, the most common AIDS-defining disease is now tuberculosis, which is by no means exclusive to HIV-positive individuals.

Another AIDS defining condition is nothing more than a laboratory result. A one-time CD4+ T cell count of less than 200 per milliliter is sufficient for a diagnosis of AIDS in the US. Interestingly, from the beginning researchers were looking for an infectious agent that was tropic for CD4+ T cells, and "HIV disease" was considered for years to be defined by the loss of such cells via direct or indirect HIV-mediated destruction. Forty years into the epidemic, there is still no agreed-upon mechanism of said depletion, and the presence of so few infected T cells rendered this assumption suspicious. Modes of destruction involving healthy T cells somehow being primed for destruction have been proposed, but never witnessed.

Furthermore, there are other laboratory anomalies often to be found in AIDS patients and HIV-positive individuals, including elevated levels of circulating antibodies of many kinds, and deficiencies in the levels of natural killer cells. Chronic inflammation is often seen as well. Interestingly, elevated levels of many types of antibodies are a known cause of so-called false positive HIV tests, which might lead the reader to wonder if the entire construction might be circular in its logic.

The question has to be asked: What would have happened if, from the early days of AIDS, we had been looking for an agent capable of causing depletion in natural killer cells and other abnormalities now known to be associated with AIDS? If we hadn't been so laser focused on CD4+ T cells, would we have found something different?

The changing face of AIDS, as well as the prevalence of certain immunological disorders and dysregulation in populations outside the risk groups, strongly suggest that we have lost our way—or that something is being concealed from the public through fraud, incompetence, or plain old self-deception. Given that the AIDS of the 1980s had changed significantly in its severity by the early 1990s (AIDS deaths began to drop between 1993–95, *before* the advent of highly active antiretroviral therapy), it would not be unreasonable to say that the "HIV disease" of the 1990s and beyond is more akin to "long haul AIDS," of necessarily decreased severity than proto-AIDS of the early days.

Given that HIV positivity is nowhere near zero, in any population,[17] including groups such as repeat blood donors who are at no known risk of AIDS, it seems entirely reasonable to assume that HIV positivity is either incidental to, or is a direct result of disease/dysfunction rather than its cause.

Consider also the prevalence of immune disorders and autoimmune illnesses that bear more than a passing resemblance to AIDS. AIDS-defining illnesses often prove to be more like autoimmunity or a very specific decline in cell-mediated immunity, rather than being similar to classical immune deficiencies from cancer chemotherapy, for example. Chronic inflammation, for example, is known to be common in AIDS patients, but inflammation is not an immune deficiency but rather closer to an immune *over*-reaction.

There are also diseases and syndromes seen outside the classical risk groups that bear more than a passing similarity to AIDS; so much so that the category of "HIV-negative AIDS" was introduced in 1993. One such striking example is myalgic encephalomyelitis, more commonly known as chronic fatigue syndrome. Another name for this disorder is "chronic fatigue immune dysfunction," and it is characterized by debilitating fatigue, susceptibility to infection, and cognitive disturbances. Additionally, it is common for ME/CFS patients to experience lymphadenopathy, night sweats, and bowel disturbances. All of these symptoms are common to AIDS as well, making ME/CFS look awfully like "non risk group, HIV-negative long haul AIDS." Inflammation and depletion of natural killer cells are commonly observed in ME/CFS as well as AIDS, but the difference is almost entirely in who gets which disease. ME/CFS appears almost as a mirror image of AIDS, being more common in women than men, and almost never to be seen in AIDS risk group populations.

Other immune disturbances that are clinically similar to AIDS include lupus and Lyme disease.

The question I will pose to close this section is the following: Does the HIV/AIDS designation exist solely to ghettoize the risk groups, so that they can be "retained in care" to take drugs that either are (in the case of TDF) or should be the subject of class action lawsuits?

If It Isn't HIV, What Is It?

AIDS is real; HIV is not, and they [old guard researchers] need to move over on the research bench so we can get some real answers.
—Liam Scheff, 2007, personal communication

The bottom line, the end point that I hope readers take away from this modest volume, is that HIV is not necessary to explain any case of AIDS. There is no case of AIDS or "long haul AIDS" that cannot be explained without resorting to pointing the finger at a retrovirus that is barely to be found in anyone, including AIDS patients, and may not even exist in the traditional way of existence attributed to other exogenous pathogens.

The best we have managed to do in forty years is to come up with the pronouncement that "U=U" (meaning that if an individual "retained in care" has undetectable viral load, their alleged infection is "untransmittable," and for which the best evidence comes from a one-page opinion piece coauthored by Anthony Fauci,[18] which admits up front the lack of clinical trial evidence to support "U = U") and medicate not only HIV-antibody-positive individuals, *but even HIV-antibody-negatives* who are not only "at risk" but merely "concerned," with chemotherapeutics with severe adverse effects for life. This is disturbing in light of the fact that official estimates consider the risk of sexual transmission per encounter to be *at most* 2 percent, and typically closer to 1 in 1000. The true value, according to official sources, is likely to be much lower as retrospective studies have found no seroconversions at all among discordant couples.

Consider also that by 1985, when AIDS was supposedly a new disease, official estimates for the prevalence of HIV-positivity were that one million Americans were HIV-positive. This figure has remained essentially the same when adjusting for population growth. The idea of a barely contagious disease spreading to every risk group in every part of the country within years, and then to stop spreading in any significant way, defies logic and certainly should have long ago belied the concept of HIV as an STI or a contagious disease.

Indeed, the *only* effective way of transmitting HIV-positivity is perinatally, from mother to child. Estimates for perinatal transmission are usually given as 20–30 percent. Paired with the knowledge that even in unmedicated people, HIV-positivity is barely (if at all) transmissible, and that the distribution of HIV-positivity is identical with respect to race and geographic location *in every risk group,* it seems that HIV-positivity indicates something far more likely to be genetically linked than an STI.

Consider again how AIDS changed dramatically between the early 1980s and ten years later, prior to the advent of the highly active antiretroviral therapy. We note that the peak of AIDS deaths occurred between 1993 and 1995. In chapter four, we will review the change in the definition of AIDS by the Centers for Disease Control and Prevention that massively expanded the pool of potential AIDS patients by including lab test results as a clinical endpoint capable of classifying a person as an AIDS patient without having any physical symptoms at all.

Indeed, it is even possible that the classification of AIDS as an *immune deficiency* is not quite accurate; AIDS patients suffer from *immune dysregulation* as evidenced by the fact that the HIV antibody tests measure, by design, excess levels of circulating antibodies *of many types*, not "HIV specific" antibodies as we have been led to believe. Additionally, in the early days of AIDS, patients were often treated successfully with high dose steroids, which are commonly thought of as *immunosuppressant*. Why would patients suffering an immune deficiency improve when given immmuno-suppressant drugs?

I will draw the reader's attention to the work of the late electron microscopist, Etienne de Harven. He was a Belgian physician and pioneer in electron microscopy, which is the technique of using an extremely high-powered microscope to see particles not visible via regular microscope. In particular, viruses, particles many times smaller than bacteria, can be seen under the electron microscope. Retroviruses are known to band at a particular density gradient in a centrifuge, and when extracted from the centrifuged mixture, can be easily seen under the electron microscope.

De Harven published in 1958 the first electron micrographs of a retrovirus, the Friend leukemia virus, found in mice. In 1960, he observed via electron microscopy that retroviral particles "bud" on the cell's outer membrane.

What is interesting about de Harven is that from the moment a retroviral cause was speculated about for AIDS to his death in 2019, he contended that this causal relationship was impossible. He pointed first to the seminal Gallo papers of 1984 and to the fact that of the only 34 percent of patients who had any trace of HIV, and that the allegedly infected cells in which the virus is meant to be replicating and therefore depleting, the host cells do not in fact become depleted but survive indefinitely.

De Harven was especially critical of the electron micrographs presented in the Gallo papers. According to de Harven, convincing electron micrographic evidence to support the isolation of a retrovirus should be twofold: one needs to show retroviral-like particles of the same size and shape in *uncultured* tissue samples; the other needs to show isolates of these objects. What the Gallo papers showed were micrographs of cultures that were stimulated by mitogens and to which were added the immune cells or plasma of AIDS patients. The micrographs of so-called "HIV isolates" that were published in *Virology* in 1997 were no more impressive, containing mostly non-viral material. In the words of de Harven himself, "The faith in retroviruses as pathogens assumed quasi-religious proportions. Since electron microscopy could not demonstrate viruses in the 1.16 bands [density gradient at which retroviruses collect] from human subjects, we forgot about microscopy and started relying on 'markers.' [. . .] When retroviruses are legion, molecular markers provide a useful approach to quantification . . . but without isolates, the use of markers is methodological nonsense. 'Markers' of what? We all know that all of the so-called 'HIV markers' are totally non-specific."

De Harven was also critical of the use of reverse transcriptase as a marker for HIV, although it is widely considered to be such. RT is the enzyme that transcribes RNA to DNA rather than the other way around as is typical. RT has been found in yeasts, insects, mammals, and umbilical cord tissues, and is by no means exclusive to HIV.

The recollections of de Harven dovetail quite nicely with the work of the Perth Group, who assert that HIV has never actually been isolated, nor proven to exist as a unique exogenous retrovirus.

Indeed, human DNA is full of retroviral particles that are often released as endogenous retroviruses at times of rapid cell growth and/or destruction. These HERVs (human endogenous retroviruses) are often to be found at elevated levels in many disease states, and have even been shown to be capable of producing pathological effects by encoding a superantigen.

The 2016 paper "Extracellular vesicles and viruses: Are they close relatives?" coauthored by none other than Robert Gallo, is quite intriguing.[19] In the abstract of this publication, the authors state the following: "Extracellular vesicles (EVs) released by various cells are small phospholipid membrane-enclosed entities that can carry mRNA. Physical and chemical characteristics of EVs, as well as their biogenesis pathways, resemble those of retroviruses. Moreover, EVs generated by virus-infected cells can incorporate viral proteins and fragments of viral RNA, being thus indistinguishable from defective retroviruses."

Further discussion of the potential role of endogenous retroviruses in the pathology of AIDS and other immunological dysfunction can be found in the work of the Perth Group as well as others. It is notable that in the early 1980s, the relative abundance of endogenous retroviruses, and of retroviral DNA in the human genome, was not well known or understood. How differently would the game have been played had we been armed with this understanding?

Indeed, attention has been drawn in recent years to the human endogenous retrovirus HERV-K18, which has been shown to encode a superantigen that can trigger immune dysregulation when activated by Epstein-Barr virus and human herpesvirus-6 (HHV6), among others.

As de la Hera et. al.[20] noted, "HERVs are genomic sequences that resulted from ancestral germ-line infections by exogenous retroviruses and therefore are transmitted in a Mendelian fashion. Increased HERV expression and antibodies to HERV antigens have been found in various autoimmune diseases."

Given this information and the analysis of Bauer that strongly implies that HIV-positivity cannot be infectious but rather behaves more like a genetically transmitted condition (recall that MTC transmission is by far the most effective means of transmitting "HIV positivity"), it seems a reasonable question to ask whether what has been identified as HIV is not, in fact, exogenous at all but may be a byproduct of a HERV with associated antibody-generating proteins. Given that HERVs are capable of inducing the expression of disease-causing superantigens, the implication of a HERV in AIDS and other immune dysfunction disease states can explain both the relatively low transmissiblity of HIV and the elevated risk of disease in populations at risk. Regardless, it remains the case that human beings are host to a large number of both endogenous and exogenous retroviruses, none of which has been shown to cause harm directly.

The initial mistake that was made in the early 1980s, in a rush to solve what was at the time the greatest medical mystery in many years, was that the scientific community very quickly "zoomed in" on the loss of CD4+ T cells as the almost exclusive defining laboratory anomaly of AIDS patients to the exclusion of almost everything else, which then led to the search for a pathogen that was attracted to said CD4+ T cells, which led to HIV and the rest is history. In my opinion, this has been a colossal failure on the part of the scientific community, not only for those suffering from AIDS or testing positive for antibody to HIV, but also to the millions of people suffering immune dysregulation in the absence of any indication of HIV-positivity. "Zooming in" on HIV ignores the many other laboratory anomalies found in AIDS patients, including but not limited to elevated antibody production, changes in the Th1 and Th2 cell populations, lymphocytopenia in general, and declines in the levels of natural killer cells. How much more would we now know had we, instead of zooming in on HIV, zoomed out on the general concept of immune dysregulation. It is certainly true that *many* HIV-negative individuals would fit the CDC's criteria for "having AIDS" if the presence of antibody to HIV were not *required* for a diagnosis of AIDS. Again, this is an indication that we would be better served by zooming out rather than zooming in.

All that HIV theory has given us are myriad failed predictions, no convincingly answered questions, and at best, a large number of people that can claim to be "virally suppressed." None of this addresses any epidemic of immune dysfunction, as it focuses *entirely* on a surrogate marker, which has not been shown to have any correlation with health. Indeed, the problem is even worse, due to the push to prescribe PrEP to even HIV-negative individuals. Instead of addressing the problem at its source, we put the band-aid of "anti HIV drugs" on the problem and hope it will go away. It has not gone away, and there are frightening hints that today's band-aid could prove to be tomorrow's Thalidomide.

The COVID crisis has shown many people that the public health bureaucrats do not necessarily have our best interests at heart. These people are not benevolent scientists with no vested interest, hidden in their ivory towers producing "the science." They are businesspeople beholden to the politically motivated granting agencies and to the pharmaceutical companies. Yes, many if not most of them have good intentions. That doesn't make them beyond questioning. It doesn't even make them right, because science should be divorced from consensus.

Unfortunately, the COVID crisis taught many of us that these supposedly benevolent public health czars and politicians are not above weaponizing a *virus* or a narrative about a disease to divide people, turn families and friends against each other, and imply that human contact is inherently dangerous and should be avoided if possible. One can only commune with similarly "good, rule followers." But this has happened before, with HIV. In some states, one can still be imprisoned for not revealing their HIV-positivity. HIV has been from the beginning an efficient way to "other," or ghettoize, certain marginalized communities, gay men, and Black Americans and Africans being the most victimized. It has become so *de rigueur* to talk about this AIDS phenomenon in terms of "risk groups" and "lifestyle choices" that most people don't even realize they are doing it anymore. This needs to stop. In order for it to stop, we need to zoom out and recognize that my quote from Liam Scheff is absolutely on the money. AIDS is real, HIV is not. As soon as the scientific community accepts this fact, as soon as we take a step back and reassess what we have learned in light of *actually* treating immune dysfunction beyond simply trying to control surrogate markers, there will be rich opportunities to get some *real* answers. The challenge we face is that in some sense, the HIV empire is too big to fail. But fail it must.

Introduction

The Paradox of the Prevalence Curve

Any book that purports to reveal and explain the many flaws, paradoxes, and examples of circular logic—and often just plain *il*logic—in the HIV=AIDS=DEATH theory should introduce the reader to one such fatal flaw straight away. And so, I present to you the paradox of the US HIV prevalence curve.[21]

Before I present the curve itself, please note that although many of the arguments presented in this narrative refer specifically to North America (and by extension, Europe, as part of the First World), essentially all of them apply to HIV and AIDS anywhere else in the world. The virological and immunological arguments I present are, of course, applicable no matter what geographic location one wants to consider. But this applies to the epidemiology as well because most of the reports we hear about HIV rates in places like Asia and Africa are simply statistical contrivances with no basis in reality.* Although it is true that the raw prevalence of HIV in sub-Saharan Africa is indeed higher than it is in North America and Europe, the fact is that in no case does HIV prevalence ever fit with AIDS incidence.

The word *curve* is actually a misnomer when it comes to describing the HIV prevalence graph shown below because as you can clearly see, with the exception of a small *drop* in case estimates in 1995, the prevalence of HIV in the US has remained, for all intents and purposes, perfectly constant since testing began in 1985 (See Figure 1).

Please note also that although the graph terminates in the year 2000, official estimates remain similar, and the latest CDC estimates for HIV prevalence state that approximately one million Americans currently test positive for HIV,[22,23] a fact that would change the graph little.

It is important as well to point out that although, yes, this curve is estimated—largely owing to the fact that because not everyone tests for HIV, we can never be sure *exactly* how many Americans truly test positive—the estimations on which this graph is based depend upon what are still very high levels of testing. HIV prevalence estimates in the US are in fact based upon more actual testing than almost any other disease testing.[17]

In contrast to the HIV prevalence curve, US AIDS cases peaked in 1993–94.[21] Although this was due, at least in part, to the expansion of the AIDS definition by the CDC in 1993, it is

---

* Although heterosexual transmission is presumed to be responsible for 70 to 80 percent of HIV infections worldwide, with the vast majority of cases occurring in Asia and sub-Saharan Africa, the actual data reported indicate the impossibility of the statement. Specifically, the transmission probabilities reported for Africa (Gray et al. 2001; Hugonnet et al., n.d.) are effectively identical those in the US (Padian et al. 1997), revealing the impossibility of a heterosexually transmitted epidemic anywhere in the world.

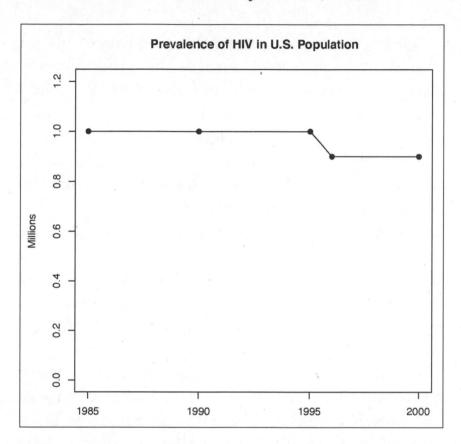

Figure 1.

clear that the AIDS epidemic is non-constant, and indeed, after increasing slowly prior to 1993, it has gradually declined up to the present day. We often hear phrases in the lay media such as "The number of AIDS cases is double what it was *x* number of years ago," which creates a false sense of alarm because it implies that *many more people are now developing AIDS than ever before.* What the media reports don't mention, however, is that the numbers given are cumulative totals, in which all new cases for a given year are added to all the cases for all the years prior to yield a running total. Of course, if you continually add up all the AIDS cases since the beginning of AIDS record keeping, it will be impossible to ever obtain a decrease.

The true numbers of annual AIDS cases, however, are not reflected by cumulative totals but rather by annual incidences. The figure above displays the estimated number of HIV-antibody-positive people in the US for each given year, and as the figure clearly conveys, this number has remained almost perfectly constant since 1985 at about one million. With a US population of about 295 million people, this amounts to only 0.4 percent of US citizens testing positive for HIV antibody.

This data should sound a clear alarm when one considers the supposed "infectious" nature of AIDS (and possibly HIV). First, if HIV is a new pathogen, then its presence should not have remained constant—it should have clearly increased according to Farr's Law, which asserts that a new contagion spreads exponentially throughout the population. More damning, however, is the following.

HIV is said to cause AIDS on average eight to ten years after infection. If HIV causes AIDS, then the incidence of AIDS should have mirrored the prevalence of HIV, only shifted eight to ten years into the future. If HIV causes AIDS, the AIDS incidence curve should be flat. This is not the case.

This discrepancy cannot be explained away by AIDS drugs because this cannot account for the sharp rise in AIDS incidence between 1987, when the first AIDS drugs were marketed, and the drop that began in 1993.

There are many more flaws in the HIV theory of AIDS, and the following pages will highlight some of the more damning of these. It should certainly be clear to anyone who was around during the 1980s that AIDS looks nothing like what it was predicted to look like twenty years ago. The growing focus on Africa—and to a lesser extent Asia—is merely a tactic to keep people supportive of AIDS, and thus maintain the funding of scientists and activists who work on AIDS, because it is clear that if we were to base our decisions upon what is happening at home, the AIDS industry would all but disappear. Instead, we remain transfixed by the notion of a deadly sexual plague decimating all of Africa and potentially decimating any of us because of our inherent human need to focus our collective fears and insecurities on a tangible, concrete threat.

AIDS has become so mired in emotion, hysteria and politics that it is no longer primarily a health issue. AIDS has been transported out of the realm of public and personal health and into a strange new world in which pronouncements by powerful government officials and ill-informed celebrities are taken as gospel, and no one even remembers when, a few years later, these pronouncements turn out to be false.

If we were to rewind the clock twenty-five years and superimpose today's beliefs about AIDS onto the landscape, it might raise a few eyebrows.

Some examples: First of all, there's the clinical latency period—the time from initial infection with HIV to the development of the syndrome AIDS. Initially, the asymptomatic phase from infection to AIDS was six months. This figure grew to a year, then five years, then ten, and now—as there remain people who remain inexplicably healthy since the mid-1980s despite alleged infection with a supposedly deadly virus—fifteen, twenty years . . . who knows?

Then there is the indisputable fact that neither AIDS nor HIV have spread like they were predicted to. The predicted heterosexual AIDS explosion never happened, and to even mention this prediction now is almost taboo as it is such an embarrassment to the AIDS establishment. As we observed from the prevalence curve, HIV has not spread at all, but rather it has remained constant in the population since its detection. The African epidemic looks suspiciously nothing like the American and European epidemic, and closer inspection reveals it likely that this African epidemic is pure fabrication.[†]

You might remember that in 1987 the CDC, via Oprah Winfrey, made the dire prediction that by 1990, one in five heterosexuals would likely be dead of AIDS. You might remember that both a vaccine and a cure were promised by 1986. You might wonder why people died so quickly on AZT, supposedly a "magic bullet." You might notice that they aren't dying so quickly on the new drugs—but then why do they look so wasted, drawn, and sick? Something's wrong here.

Scratching the surface just a little bit more, one uncovers many more problems than just some bad drugs and some clearly faulty predictions. The problems range from the fact that no one really understands how HIV actually works—or even, for that matter, what HIV really is—to the paradox of how a disease could cause both vastly different epidemiologies and symptomatic presentations in the First and Third Worlds.

[†]   African AIDS is diagnosed differently from AIDS anywhere else in the world. The so-called Bangui definition, arrived at in 1985 at a WHO meeting in Bangui, Central African Republic, consists of a set of symptoms with *no test for HIV antibodies necessary.* These symptoms are easily confused with those of tuberculosis, malaria, dysentery, cholera, and other common African diseases. Furthermore, in places where HIV testing is available, the criteria for a positive HIV test are the least stringent of any in the world, dramatically increasing the likelihood of cross-reactivity, particularly in a place where cross-reacting agents are common. Finally, estimates of the HIV prevalence in Africa such as those trumpeted in the world media are derived from blood tests given to pregnant women at antenatal clinics. What happens is that pregnant women are tested for syphilis as part of routine prenatal care, and some of the blood samples that are left behind are anonymously given a single ELISA antibody test. The results of these tests are then extrapolated to the general population via computer simulation. The problems with this approach are many and include the fact that pregnancy itself is a source of false positives, compounded by the fact that a single ELISA test will give an unacceptably high number of false positives.

As has been said by others, there are no paradoxes in nature, only flawed hypotheses.[24] Questions about HIV and AIDS have been raised since HIV was first discovered, and as the years pass, the questions accumulate but remain largely unanswered. Any such theory—one that cannot even answer questions for which it was put forth—should be looked at very critically.

CHAPTER 1

How I Came to Change My Mind

Scientists have been criticizing the HIV causes AIDS paradigm for over thirty years now. What makes me any different?

My chosen career has developed around the HIV model of AIDS. I received my PhD in 2002 for my work constructing mathematical models of the immunological aspects of HIV infection, a field of study I entered in 1996. Just ten years later, it might seem early for me to be looking back on and seriously reconsidering my chosen field, yet here I am.

My work as a mathematical biologist has been built in large part on the paradigm that HIV causes AIDS, and I have since come to realize that there is good evidence that the entire basis for this theory is wrong. AIDS, it seems, is not a disease so much as a socio-political construct that few people understand and even fewer question. The issue of causation, in particular, has become beyond question—even to bring it up is deemed irresponsible.

Why have we as a society been so quick to accept a theory for which so little solid evidence exists? Why do we take proclamations by government institutions like the NIH and the CDC, via newscasters and talk show hosts, entirely on faith? The average citizen has no idea how weak the connection really is between HIV and AIDS, and this is the manner in which scientifically insupportable phrases like "the AIDS virus" or "an AIDS test" have become part of the common vernacular despite no evidence for their accuracy.

I have come to the conclusion that massive scientific, governmental, and societal acceptance of the HIV causes AIDS model has little to do with any real evidence implicating HIV. The paradigm has been supported from the beginning by government institutions that, perhaps inadvertently, encourage poor-quality scientific research standards. But the problem is even more complex than that. There is something truly bizarre about the fact that the announcement of the discovery of the causative agent of AIDS—via press conference, no less—was immediately accepted by scientists and citizens alike before any supporting evidence had been published or critiqued in the scientific literature. Although I believe that the decline in scientific standards is the major reason HIV researchers seem to suffer from tunnel vision and some sort of collective amnesia that enables them to consider no other cause for the complex phenomenon of immune deficiency other than a single virus, as well as to conveniently "forget" every few years when they announce a new and exciting discovery that will "explain everything" that a similarly new and exciting discovery from a few years back is now shown to be wrong, there are more subtle forces at work here. The sociological reasons behind society's immediate acceptance of the HIV theory are profound and far-reaching, and I will address these later.

As a child, I felt terrorized by the specter of AIDS. When it was announced in 1984 that the cause of AIDS had been found in a retrovirus that came to be known as HIV, there was a palpable panic. My own family was immediately affected by this panic because my mother had had several blood transfusions in the early eighties as a result of three late miscarriages she had experienced. In the early days, we feared mosquito bites, kissing, and public toilet seats. I can still recall the panic I felt after looking up in a public restroom and seeing some graffiti that read: "Do you have AIDS yet? If not, sit on this toilet seat."

But as a teenager, I noticed that within a few short years, people stopped distinguishing between those who were "HIV-positive" and those who actually had AIDS, beginning to assume they were the same thing. I was no expert in the field by any means, but I paid attention to the news and have always had an interest in medicine, and I could not see the defining event that caused people to accept the change from HIV as "the virus associated with AIDS" to "the virus that causes AIDS." I remember people referred to Magic Johnson as "having AIDS" and I objected, purely on the basis of logic, "No, he's *HIV-positive*. That's not the same thing."

However, years passed, and I simply assumed that HIV did cause AIDS, that more and more people were going to get sick and die, but that it was possible that some HIV-positives were simply carriers who might never get sick. I certainly heard enough stories about long-term, AIDS-drug-free survivors to plant a seed of doubt in my mind that HIV did not *always* lead to AIDS.

One of the reasons that I chose to write a master's thesis on mathematical models of HIV infection was my curiosity about this disease, and I figured this would be an excellent way to read as much of the medical literature as possible and to start getting some answers. Little did I know, as I completed my master's degree and continued to write a PhD dissertation on the same subject, that what I would learn would go a long way toward explaining why I'd always been so confused about AIDS.

CHAPTER 2

Science Sold Out

AIDS is said to be caused principally by the HIV-mediated destruction of CD4+ T cells. The first conundrum I encountered was the lack of agreement on, or evidence for, *any* mechanism by which HIV supposedly caused this cell death. The second problem, less troubling on a purely virological level, but much more disturbing in light of scientific standards, was that papers on the molecular biology of HIV seemed to have a very short shelf life –they go out of date very quickly. In mathematics a journal article takes a significant amount of time to write and at least several months to go through the review process. By the time a paper appears in print, it may well be years from the time the work was first started. On several occasions I submitted papers with fairly recent references regarding various aspects of HIV's molecular biology, only to be answered with criticism from a reviewer that some of these references were now "out of date." Sometimes the references were only two or three years old. I later discovered that this is a common occurrence in HIV research. Science, of course, is meant to be self-correcting, but it seems to be endemic in HIV research that, rather than continually building on an accumulated body of secure knowledge with only occasional missteps, the bulk of the structure gets knocked down every three to four years, replaced by yet another hypothesis, standard of care, or definition of what, exactly, AIDS really is. This new structure eventually gets knocked down in the same fashion.

Even more disturbing is the fact that HIV researchers continually claim that certain papers' results are out of date, yet have absolutely no hesitation in citing the entire body of scientific research on HIV as massive overwhelming evidence in favor of HIV. They can't have it both ways, yet this is exactly what they try to do.

There are further problems with the scientific method surrounding HIV and AIDS, which shall be dealt with in later chapters. Among the major problems are the circumstances surrounding the publication of the initial papers by Robert Gallo's group that appeared in the journal *Science* following the historic 1984 press conference;[25] continuing difficulties in demonstrating a cell-killing role for HIV; continuing problems with (and an apparent lack of interest in) properly designating HIV as an exogenous retrovirus; and, possibly worst of all, the astounding lack of specificity, standardization, and reproducibility of the HIV antibody and viral load tests.

The question still remains: How could science have gone so far astray? Why did the scientific community accept the HIV hypothesis so readily before any papers were published to support it? And how has this belief persisted so long despite results becoming "outdated" every few years? Why is there such disagreement between dissenting and orthodox scientists regarding the standards to which such crucial cornerstones as isolation procedures and antibody testing should adhere? How could scientists have so readily allowed their research to settle into one narrow, *unproven* channel of investigation? It's been over twenty (thirty) years—surely, if something was wrong with the theory, this fact would have been discovered. Corrective action would have been taken, and a "diverse portfolio of research direction" would have been explored.[26]

The answer to these questions is twofold. The easy part of this answer is that, in point of fact, there are literally thousands of people, many of whom are credentialed doctors and scientists, who have insisted for many years that AIDS researchers have been entirely on the wrong path, or at the very least, have closed off legitimate lines of inquiry. There are many scientists who do not ascribe a pathogenic role to HIV at all, and yet more who contend that HIV alone is not the primary cause of AIDS. The latter include scientists such as Gordon Stewart, Robert Root-Bernstein, Joseph Sonnabend, Michael Lange, and Harry Rubin.

The most well-known of the scientists who believe that HIV is harmless is undoubtedly Peter Duesberg, who is often cited as having been discredited despite the fact that there is no record of this "discrediting" anywhere in the scientific literature. By contrast, Duesberg has provided the most exhaustive critique to date of all the reasons HIV cannot possibly cause AIDS, and his criticisms have never been refuted anywhere in the peer-reviewed literature. The only "refutations" to Duesberg's arguments can be found in anonymously authored, non-peer-reviewed documents such as the NIH publication "The Evidence That HIV Causes AIDS"[27] and the Durban Declaration,[28] both of which have been thoroughly rebutted themselves.[29]

Perhaps just as telling as Duesberg's experience is the fact that the inventor of the polymerase chain reaction (PCR)– to date *the* method of choice for quantifying HIV viral load—Nobel laureate Kary Mullis, states categorically that quantitative PCR is invalid and should absolutely not be used for viral load testing.

The renowned expert electron microscopist Dr. Etienne de Harven became frustrated at the very onset of the HIV paradigm. He shares the distinction of having produced the first electron micrograph of a retrovirus (the Friend leukemia virus). Since the beginning, de Harven has been skeptical not only that HIV could cause any disease but, further, that HIV has ever been properly isolated. He was at the time, and remained until his death, highly critical of all viral isolation procedures employed by HIV researchers. He contends that retrovirologists began using "shortcut," indirect methods not because of their increased efficiency, but because they couldn't get the results they wanted using the standard methods.[30]

Dr. Rodney Richards, a chemist who worked for the company AmGen developing the first HIV antibody tests, contends that HIV has never been properly isolated and that the antibody tests are at best measuring a condition called *hypergammagloulinemia*, a mouthful of a word that simply means having too many antibodies to too many things.

Dr. David Rasnick, who received his PhD in biochemistry for studying human proteases and holds several patents on protease inhibitors for various human diseases, has been highly critical of the HIV hypothesis since 1985. Furthermore, he strongly contends that the AIDS era has rendered clinical trial standards so low as to be nearly nonexistent.

John Lauritsen, a gay journalist and historian, has doubted the HIV hypothesis since its inception and has been extremely vocal about the incredible disservice a virus-only theory of AIDS has done to the gay community. His background in statistical survey research led to his extreme frustration with the lack of standards in epidemiological research and clinical trials. His exposé of the fraud and astonishing lack of standards that affect HIV clinical trials, in particular those that led to the initial approval of the drug AZT, are documented in his book *Poison by Prescription: The AZT story*.

To put it plainly, HIV science has sold out to the epidemic of low standards that is infecting all of academic scientific research.

At the time of this writing, I had been employed at the faculty level in university academia for four years, and prior to that I spent a total of four years doing graduate-level research. (The gap perceived by my having stated that I first began ten years before owes to the fact that following my master's degree I spent two years working in industry.) I have also observed my father's employment circumstances and academic research experience as a professor in the physical sciences. Over the years, I have had plenty of opportunity to see exactly how research expectations affect the quality of work we produce. It is clear to me that the pressure to obtain big government grants and to publish as many papers as possible is not necessarily helping the advancement of science. Rather, academics (young ones, in particular) are pressured to choose projects that can be completed quickly and easily, so they can increase their publication list as fast as possible. As a result, quality suffers.

This lowering of scientific standards and critical thinking has been apparent in many aspects of research for some time, and it is now beginning to infiltrate the classroom—in the textbooks and the undergraduate curriculum. It is germane at this point to indicate that many of the common arguments presented in response to the queries of HIV skeptics are essentially some form of appeal to the use of low standards. (For example, "You don't need a reference that HIV causes AIDS," "The fact that HIV and AIDS are so well correlated indicates that it must be the cause," "HIV is a new virus, and new viruses will meet new standards," "Koch's postulates are outdated and don't apply in this day and age," "We don't need to worry about the actual infectious virus, viral markers should suffice," or "Real scientists do experiments; they don't write review articles on the literature.") All of these observations are eloquently summed up by the mathematician Mark Craddock:

> Science is about making observations and trying to fit them into a theoretical framework. Having the theoretical framework allows us to make predictions about phenomena that we can then test. HIV "science" long ago set off on a different path . . . People who ask simple, straightforward questions are labelled as loonies who are dangerous to public health.[31]

It is this decline in scientific standards that I point to when I am asked how so many scientists and doctors could be so wrong. Given the current research atmosphere, it was almost inevitable that a very significant scientific mistake was going to be made.

CHAPTER 3

Science by Consensus

If the AIDS establishment is so convinced of the validity of what they say, they should have no fear of a public, adjudicated debate between the major orthodox and dissenting scientists and the scrutiny of such a debate by the scientific community. Yet all the major AIDS researchers have avoided such a public debate, either by claiming that the "overwhelming scientific consensus" makes such a debate superfluous, or by saying that they are "too busy saving lives." Consider the result of the 1988 *Science* fight, to date the only such debate:

> After the "Policy Forum" appeared, Peter all but begged
> Dan to sanction another round, to no avail. And so
> just when it was getting good, the bout was declared a

technical draw on an inexplicable and non-appealable decision of commissioner Koshland. There was never to be a rematch. The failure to extend the discussion in the pages of *Science* was significant. Most scientists have neither time nor inclination to follow specialist literature in fields outside their own. They depend, consequently, on journals like *Science* and *Nature* to tell them what is considered important. Having read, as best they could at the time, the arguments of the Policy Forum, and then seeing nothing more than vulgar anti-Duesberg editorials in the scientific press and worse in the popular media, even a partially persuaded nonspecialist could and would eventually concur with the "overwhelming evidence" of Team Virus, although it has become even less overwhelming now than it was in 1988.[32]

In place of public debate, politically motivated documents such as the Durban Declaration remain the establishment's standard response to dissenting voices. Even a cursory reading of this document reveals it to be a statement of faith, designed to divert attention from dissenters at the very moment when they were threatening to expose the orthodoxy in South Africa in 2000. The Durban Declaration was signed by over five thousand "PhD researchers," which would lead one to assume that the signatories had at least familiarized themselves with the orthodox and dissident literature on HIV and AIDS. This is entirely misleading, as an email which went out as an attachment to the solicitation to sign the declaration included the following statement: "Many of you will say that HIV and AIDS is not your area, but by now you have heard enough of the arguments."[32] There is nothing scientific about the Durban Declaration—it is quite obviously a piece of propaganda somehow made authoritative by the thousands of signatures attached to it.

But science is not a democracy. As much as we would like to be able to mold our results and discoveries to fit hypotheses we would like to see proven, this is not how science should proceed. If our hypotheses fail to explain and predict, we should consider other ideas.

Until such a time as a causal role for HIV in the etiology of AIDS is decisively proven or disproven, we can only rely on the available evidence for policy and public health decisions. Furthermore, this evidence should *not* be gathered and formulated within the framework of the HIV hypothesis. Due to the current practice of discrimination against HIV-positives, as well as the apparent lack of any benefit of anti-HIV drugs, a causal role should *not* be assumed until proven, but this is exactly what has happened.

In order to truly understand how the HIV/AIDS connection became nearly universally accepted *without question*, one must revisit the early days of AIDS and the discovery of HIV. I will discuss the changing face of AIDS itself in a later chapter, so for the time being, let us consider the original evidence for HIV as given by one of its discoverers.

The first scientific papers claiming a definite causal role for HIV were published May 5, 1984, in the esteemed journal *Science*. Robert Gallo, late of the NIH, and his chief secondary collaborator, Mikulas Popovic, published four papers describing the detection of HIV in a proportion of AIDS patients and the details of how HIV was detected.[7] It is amazing that in the paper purporting to have *frequently* detected HIV in AIDS patients, actual HIV could be detected in only twenty-six out of seventy-two AIDS patients and in eighteen out of twenty-one pre-AIDS patients (pre-AIDS is an obsolete term that was used to describe a collection of symptoms including persistent fever, weight loss, and generalized lymphadenopathy). Gallo claimed that the reason for such a low frequency of detection (in spite of the title using the word *frequent*) was probably due to "sample contamination." It was later determined that his samples were indeed contaminated with mold, but one wonders how it is possible to come to such fundamental scientific conclusions using contaminated evidence!

Regardless, it seems strange that finding HIV in fewer than half of AIDS and pre-AIDS patients would ever qualify a virus for a pathogenic role, and indeed in the scientific papers Gallo's team avoided using any absolute terms to indicate causation. However, he *did* use such words in the press conference that was held before the publication of these papers. By the time the supporting papers were published, the lay press had all but declared HIV to be "the AIDS virus," and debate in the scientific arena was effectively stopped.

It was sometime in 1985 that HIV mysteriously went from "the virus associated with AIDS" to "the virus that causes AIDS," squelching debate in the scientific arena. What changed? What happened to make scientists come to such certainty? If you look at the actual papers, you'll see quite clearly that the answer is: nothing.

However, the AIDS machine kept going, and the questions of dissenting scientists were rarely acknowledged, let alone answered. One of the major problems with the HIV theory has always been that very little HIV can be found in the blood of AIDS patients and, in spite of claims to the contrary, there is no "massive covert infection" to be found in the lymph nodes, either.[33–35] How could a virus appearing at concentrations of one to ten infectious particles per milliliter—and sometimes unable to be found at all[7,36]—be considered pathogenic?

In 1995, two papers were published in the journal *Nature* that supposedly answered this question once and for all.[9,10] These papers made popular the "hit hard, hit early" and Highly Active Antiretroviral Therapy (HAART) treatment strategies, as well as the concept of viral load testing as a measure of treatment success. One of the authors, David Ho, was named *Time* magazine's "Man of the Year" in 1996. The papers have since been thoroughly discredited on both immunological and mathematical grounds.[31,37,38]

The mathematical models used in these papers claimed to show that HIV replicated furiously from day one, in contrast to earlier evidence suggesting it to be quite inactive.[33,39] Even now, few people are aware that these conclusions were based on very poorly constructed mathematical models. If analyzed properly, the models predict the onset of AIDS within *weeks* or *months* after HIV infection, *before* antiviral immunity as evidenced by the appearance of antibodies.[31] To make matters worse, the statistical analyses were very poorly done and the graphs were presented in such a way as to lead the reader to believe something different from what the data supported. Yet these papers were lauded at the time as groundbreaking and even "brilliant," leading to a "new mathematical understanding of how the immune system works," according to the former editor of *Nature*. In an editorial appearing in the very same issue, Sir John Maddox, the editor in chief of *Nature*, presented the papers as evidence once and for all that this HIV hypothesis was correct and that dissidents, most particularly Peter Duesberg, were wrong. Maddox even went so far as to say that, in light of the evidence presented in the Ho/Wei papers, "Now may be the time for [the Duesbergs of the world] to recant."

This example illustrates a central flaw in the HIV theory. The vast majority of the literature I've read uses what is known as circular logic—you assume that something will happen, and then you mold the definitions, models, experiments, and results to support that conclusion. Craddock describes a typical example of circular logic in the Wei paper:

> They are trying to estimate viral production rates by measuring viral load at different times and trying to fit the numbers to their formula for free virus. But if their formula is wrong, then their estimates for viral production will be wrong too.[31]

Such tactics, *by definition*, are excellent at maintaining the facade of a near-perfect correlation between HIV and AIDS, and of providing seemingly convincing explanations of HIV pathogenesis. But the resultant science does little to expand our actual understanding.

As has been indicated, the Ho/Wei papers have been essentially debunked by both establishment and dissenting researchers on biological as well as mathematical grounds; they are now acknowledged to be wrong by the scientific community, and it remains a mystery how they were ever able to pass peer review in the first place. It is often asked, "Why should we care at this point? Those papers are eleven years old; our understanding has progressed since then." The short answer is that viral load and combination therapies are used to this day, despite the fact that their original justification was based on these incorrect papers. Although current therapeutic regimens have been scaled back from the "hit hard, hit early" dogma that was popular ten years ago, the fact remains that a large population of people have been, and continue to be, treated on the basis of a theory that is fundamentally unsupportable.

Yet there is another answer to this question which is even more fundamental. It is a curious fact that few HIV researchers seem to be bothered by the events surrounding the Ho/Wei papers. You might imagine that people may care at this point because of concern over the integrity of science. You might imagine that people might feel an urge to discuss the manner in which the papers got published and whether other such mistakes have happened since that time. You might imagine that the failure of the peer-review process to detect such patently inept research would send off alarm bells within the HIV-research community.

You would be wrong.

HIV researchers know the Ho/Wei papers are wrong, yet they continue along the clinical path charted by the papers. They know that the quantitative use of PCR has never been validated, yet they continue to use viral load to make clinical decisions. They know that the history of HIV/AIDS is littered with documented cases of fraud, incompetence, and poor-quality research, yet they find it almost impossible that this could be happening in the present moment. They know their predictions have never panned out, yet they keep inventing mysterious mechanisms for HIV pathogenesis. They know many therapies of the past are now acknowledged to be mistakes (AZT monotherapy, "hit hard, hit early"), yet they never imagine that their current therapies (the ever-growing list of combination therapies) might one day be acknowledged as mistakes themselves.

It's time for them to wake up.

CHAPTER 4

What Is "AIDS"?

What we now know as "AIDS" bears little resemblance to the original cases of AIDS, as observed in New York City, Los Angeles, and San Francisco in 1981. The *original* definition of AIDS was based upon the observation of very rare opportunistic infections in previously healthy homosexual men. This list of opportunistic infections included Kaposi's sarcoma (although it is highly debatable whether KS has anything at all to do with immune suppression), *Pneumocystis carinii* pneumonia, cytomegalovirus (CMV) infection, and severe candidiasis.[40] The status of "HIV-positive" had nothing to do with a diagnosis of AIDS prior to 1984, as HIV had yet to be identified.

It is worth noting that AIDS was *not* originally conceived as a specific disease. The definition was developed as a surveillance tool to assist clinicians and epidemiologists in identifying and controlling this strange new syndrome. It remains a matter largely hidden from the public that the first cases of AIDS did not suddenly arrive all at once, but rather were sought out by an assistant professor of immunology at UCLA Medical Center named Michael Gottlieb in 1981. After searching hospitals in Los Angeles for gay men suffering from opportunistic infections, he managed to find five.[41] Upon measuring their T-cells, a subset of the immune system, he found that in all five men they were depleted. What is quite curious about this discovery is the technology to count T-cells had only just been perfected.

The acronym AIDS was introduced to replace the previously used pejorative term GRID (Gay-Related Immune Deficiency). Regardless, AIDS remains to this day a government-defined *syndrome* with, simultaneously, no specific clinical symptoms of its own yet a myriad of indirect illnesses and symptoms supposedly "caused" by the immune suppression—really quite a clever idea, since essentially everything is a symptom.

A clinical syndrome is useful when initially attempting to better understand what might be the causative agent of said syndrome. Plainly speaking, one designates a syndrome *before* one has any knowledge of the precise molecular mechanism of pathogenesis underlying the set of symptoms. Defining the clinical syndrome enables public health authorities and physicians to narrow the scope of their investigation to factors common to all those people in the epidemiological cohort among which the syndrome is manifest. A clinical syndrome is useful when it illuminates a causative agent of a disease, and this identification ideally has the effect of narrowing the scope of the clinical syndrome. That is, as we know more about what causes the syndrome, the number of symptoms under the syndrome umbrella should become smaller as we identify and throw out those that clearly do not fit the pattern.

AIDS is peculiar historically in that the definition of the syndrome actually became *more* expansive after the alleged causative agent was identified. This is contrary to all logic and counter to the reasoning that underlies the existence and usefulness of clinical syndromes in the first place. Moreover, these expansions make it very difficult to properly analyze epidemiological data. As the definition expanded and as it became more and more clear that HIV did not do what it was purported to do—that is, kill CD4+ T-cells by any detectable method—researchers began to invent more and more convoluted explanations for why their theory was correct. The logical, scientific thing to have done would have been to notice that the original disease designation did not accurately identify the causative agent or agents and, rather than changing the syndrome, throw out the supposed causative agent(s) and find one that explained the observations better. As we know, this has not happened.

Even a diagnosis of HIV-positive accompanied by no clinical symptoms at all can result in an individual's inclusion under the umbrella of AIDS, which flies in the face of the very reason for the designation of a *syndrome* as a set of clinical *symptoms*. In another major lapse of logic, the classification of HIV-free AIDS, "Idiopathic CD4+ Lymphocytopenia" or ICL for short, was introduced in 1993 to actually *exclude* from the AIDS designation people who were free of any trace of HIV but still had *symptoms that would ordinarily result in their being classified as having the syndrome AIDS.*[42]

One important feature of the original classification of AIDS was its distinction as occurring in "previously healthy" homosexuals. While recent reports have cast doubt on the presumption that these original AIDS patients were, in fact, previously healthy at all,[43] this distinction raises the question of why hemophiliacs were *ever* considered AIDS patients. It is well known that the immune system does not operate normally in hemophiliacs, and that clotting factor (Factor VIII) therapy is itself immunosuppressive.[44] Furthermore, hemophiliac AIDS patients experienced clinical disease presentations very different from those among other risk groups;[45] for example, candidiasis being very common but Kaposi's sarcoma virtually unseen.

The continual redefinitions of AIDS have resulted in a syndrome today whose clinical manifestation is very different from that seen in the original AIDS cases or the early 1980s. Some of the conditions listed are not even caused by immune deficiency, whereas others are clearly politically motivated, such as the 1993 inclusion of invasive cervical cancer. One can only presume that this disease was added to correct the disparity between male and female AIDS numbers, as there is little basis for including as "AIDS-defining" a cancer that is relatively common among women with no evidence of immune suppression whatsoever. After this addition, the media began issuing alarming statements such as "women are the fastest growing group of people with AIDS," conveniently neglecting to mention that the increases were simply small percentage differences and in some cases actually indicated a *decrease* in overall incidence.

Perhaps the most egregious addition was the inclusion of low T-cell numbers as qualifying a person for an AIDS diagnosis. This change came about in 1993 and resulted in the number of reported AIDS cases more than doubling overnight. The rationale for this change was as follows: the immune suppression observed in AIDS patients could be quantified by counting the number of CD4+ T-cells per cubic millimeter of blood. CD4+ T-cells are those cells for which HIV possesses a receptor, and it has been stated that the normal level of CD4+ T-cells per cubic millimeter of blood in a healthy individual is about one thousand. However, it is also well established that these counts can vary *dramatically* among healthy individuals and even within the same individual under conditions as severe as illness or drug use, or as mild as over-exercise or simply taking the measurements at different times of day.[46–48] (CD4+ T-cell counts are subject to diurnal variation, similar to variations in appetite and energy level.)

Mathematically speaking, the figure one thousand cells per cubic millimeter is a *mean* value, as average. However, the amount of variance about that average is quite high, even among the general population. The studies that do exist regarding low T-cell counts in HIV-negative patients reveal that this anomaly is common among people with infectious mononucleosis, chronic illnesses other than HIV, and even among highly trained athletes.[49] Furthermore, unusually high levels of T-cells do not generally indicate health but rather an inflammatory process in the body, such as allergies or an autoimmune condition that would cause the T-cell population to remain on "high alert."

Mainstream AIDS consensus generally holds that a CD4+ count under five hundred refers to definite immune suppression (whatever that means) and a CD4+ count under two hundred qualifies a person for a diagnosis of AIDS, even in the absence of clinical symptoms.[42] Another important aspect of the "low T-cell count AIDS" definition is that the figure two hundred refers not to an average count, nor even to the most recent T-cell count, but rather to the *lowest count ever measured*. The "low T-cell count AIDS" classification is significant in part because, given the dramatic variation possible in T-cell counts within a single person, one can almost guarantee that at some point an unmedicated person will experience a low T-cell count[*] if enough measurements are taken over time, *regardless of their HIV status.*

Beyond diagnosing hundreds of thousands of Americans[†] with a deadly disease on the basis of *no clinical disease at all*, the definition change served to create the illusion that new anti-HIV therapies were dramatically lowering the number of AIDS deaths in the early 1990s. The orthodoxy has done nothing to correct that impression. The effect of introducing an entire class of "healthy AIDS patients" was, first of all, to more than double the actual number of AIDS cases and, secondly, to drastically decrease the number of those patients who actually died. It doesn't take a trained pathologist to recognize that if a person is not experiencing any illness, they are much less likely to die of any illness anytime soon. Thus, the proportion of AIDS cases that resulted in death experienced a large drop in 1993–94, which the orthodoxy and the mass media were more than happy to portray as decreased mortality thanks to protease inhibitors. However, protease inhibitors were not even generally available to AIDS patients until 1996, over two years after the decline in the death rate began. In spite of the fact that there is little or no official evidence that HIV protease inhibitors extend life or decrease morbidity, they have been hailed as magic cure-alls. All one has to do is examine the disclaimers on the package inserts for any anti-HIV medication to realize that *none* of them have been shown to prolong life; that *all* of them cause debilitating side effects, some of which are indistinguishable

---

[*]   Medication increases T-cell count almost immediately not because HIV has been attacked so effectively but because, in any person, artificial chemical stimulation produces an effect called hysteresis, which means that the immune response surges to attack the chemical invader, creating an initial, and not necessarily beneficial or even meaningful, increase in T-cells.

[†]   Currently, most countries do not use the low T-cell definition of AIDS. Canada and most of Europe do not.

from the symptoms of AIDS itself; that none of them, with the exception of AZT in the disastrous clinical trials whose fraud has been thoroughly documented,[50] has been tested in placebo-controlled clinical trials; and that some of them have not even been tested in clinical trials at all.

The many stories of AIDS patients rising from their deathbeds to a renewal of good health and vitality are just that –stories. Such stories, however, have been interpreted as a major thorn in the side of the dissenting argument. Since anti-HIV drugs stop AIDS, HIV must cause AIDS—right?

It is worth noting at the outset that there are still no significant studies that actually demonstrate the statement that "anti-HIV drugs stop AIDS." There is simply no evidence, and this conclusion appears to have been reached as a matter of pure faith rather than being based on any solid science. The majority of evidence supporting the statement that "anti-HIV drugs stop AIDS" falls into two broad categories: people who were never sick in the first place and still aren't sick,‡ and people who were really quite ill indeed and experienced some improvement following the initiation of therapy.[51] A third category consists of people who die too quickly from the adverse effects of the drugs to ever develop AIDS.[52–54]

It constantly amazes me that HIV researchers, and HIV-drug manufacturers, can honestly and with a straight face state that since someone *who was healthy when they started therapy* happened to stay healthy for some time on the drugs, that this is some sort of credit to the medications. Since the new dosages of nucleoside analogue drugs and protease inhibitors are much lower than the massive doses of AZT that were given in the late 1980s, and that

---

‡   See http://healtoronto.com/rrsurvival.html

undoubtedly caused the deaths of many, it stands to reason that patients will not get sick *because of the drugs themselves* quite as quickly as they did fifteen years ago. So healthy people stay healthy for a while, and this is credited to the drugs—but there is no evidence to say that they would not have remained healthy even if they never took any medication at all. This is due to the fact that clinical trials of "anti-HIV" drugs rarely if ever use placebo controls, so there is no way to determine whether, for example, nevirapine is better than nothing. Trials are always in the form "AZT vs. nepiravine," and activists and researchers alike defend this fundamentally unscientific notion by saying that denying toxic drugs to HIV-positives is "unethical."

On the other hand, a person who is really quite sick and is experiencing opportunistic infections prior to beginning a regimen of antiretroviral therapy$ is likely to experience a temporary reprieve for some very logical reasons. Reverse transcriptase inhibitors are nonspecific cell killers and attack all growing cells. They will naturally attack those cells that are dividing the fastest, such as bacteria or fungi that are causing an acute illness. As a result, opportunistic infections are fairly efficiently killed by these drugs. The same is true for the protease inhibitors. Although the inhibitors are claimed to be specific to the HIV proteases, they are not *completely* specific and in the doses taken by HIV-positives they have the capacity to interfere with many non-HIV proteases. These include the proteases required for replication of bacteria, viruses, and other microbes. As one example, it has been demonstrated

§   It is worth noting that there is no such thing as an "antiviral" drug. Drugs classified as "antiviral" in general work by changing the dynamics of the host cell to make the cell inhospitable to viral replication. There is no mechanism of drug action that can eliminate viruses from the body, and this problem is further compounded with retroviruses since the retroviral DNA is incorporated into the host cell's genome and remains a part of the host for life.

that protease inhibitors appear to be particularly effective at controlling *Candida*[55] and *Pneumocystis.*[51]

Putting aside all potential nonspecific benefits of anti-HIV drugs, the fact remains that the risks appear to far outweigh these supposed benefits. Simply consider that the annual mortality rate of North American HIV-positives who were treated with anti-HIV drugs—between 6.7 and 8.8 percent—is much higher than the estimated 1 to 2 percent global mortality rate of HIV-positives *if all AIDS cases were fatal in a given year.*[24]

It should also give us pause to note that if these drugs were truly HIV-specific, then one drug should suffice, rather than combinations of three or four of them. Mainstream researchers argue that the high mutation rate of HIV necessitates that we "confuse" or "trick" the virus with many different medications. However, this is a ridiculous assertion, as it is simply impossible for any retroviral entity to mutate that much and remain viable. (The influenza viruses, by contrast, have a segmented chromosome and are capable of mutating by recombination, or rearrangement of their genes. HIV, like other retroviruses, has only approximately nine thousand nucleotides and as such is incapable of mutation by any method other than transcription error. Such transcription errors would be expected to quickly lead to mutations that render new virus particles noninfectious.) Also, if these drugs were truly HIV-specific, much smaller doses would be necessary than those that are currently prescribed.

A rather curious addition was made to the list of AIDS-defining diseases recently. it is named Immune Reconstitution Syndrome (IRIS or simply IRS), and it consists of the development of opportunistic infections while being treated with antiretroviral therapy. Official dogma states that as the immune system is gaining strength, it becomes confused and this enables AIDS-defining opportunistic infections to take hold. In reality, it seems to be just another attempt to explain away the fact that clearly the medications are not working as they were intended—just like the invention of ICL in 1993 was a convenient way to sweep all the HIV-free AIDS cases under the rug.

Consider also the fact that the leading cause of death among medicated HIV-positives is no longer even an AIDS-defining disease at all, but liver failure, a well-documented adverse effect of protease inhibitors. Amazingly, some people seem to think that's a good thing, as evidenced by the following comment by a blogger on LibertyPost.org, in response to an article I wrote:

> And worse, she claims that protease inhibitors are killing HIV patients, "And the leading cause of deaths in HIV-positives in the last few years has been liver failure, not an AIDS-defining disease in any way, but rather an acknowledged side effect of protease inhibitors, which asymptomatic individuals take in massive daily doses, for years," when that's exactly what you would hope for (mortality drastically decreasing to the point that more deaths were the result of side effects) if protease inhibitors were in fact EFFECTIVE treatments for AIDS. (Posted March 3, 2006)[56]

Another important—and really very shocking—fact is that in some states and countries, you don't have to die of an AIDS-defining illness to die of AIDS. In Massachusetts, for example, all deaths among HIV-positives are counted as AIDS deaths, and this happens if the person died of liver failure, a heart attack, suicide, drowning, CMV infection, or a car accident, *or anything else*, AIDS-related or not.[57]

If it weren't bad enough that perfectly healthy asymptomatic individuals who just happen to test positive for some arguably nonspecific antibodies are pressured to begin regimens of just such drugs without being given adequate information about side effects, infants and children often have no choice at all in the matter. At least adults have the opportunity to decline such medicine and are capable of gathering sufficient information to make an informed decision—although admittedly, much of the vital information regarding toxicity is not readily available from mainstream sources. Infants born to HIV-positive mothers are in many states forced to undergo antiretroviral therapy, and since only a few drugs have been approved for children, the drugs administered are usually among the most toxic, AZT and nevirapine being foremost. Oftentimes this drug regimen begins before the baby is born, in certain cases against the wishes of the mother, and continues throughout childhood. A particularly shocking example of the lengths to which HIV-treatment activists will go to ensure no child left behind in their quest to medicate at any cost is the forced drug trials that HIV-positive children underwent in New York City's Incarnation Children's Center (ICC) recently. Investigative journalist Liam Scheff uncovered the fact that children were being force-fed HIV drugs against their will while in the custody of ICC and that if the children refused to take drugs orally, a tube was inserted into their stomach to render any treatment noncompliance impossible.[3] This atrocity was further examined in a BBC documentary, *Guinea Pig Kids*, which was based on Scheff's work and aired in Europe, but not in the US

New CDC recommendations encourage *all* pregnant women to be tested for HIV antibodies, regardless of risk. This may seem a commonsense guideline until the evidence is examined more closely. One of the immediate problems is that pregnancy itself is an admitted common cause of false positives on the HIV test,[58–62] so there is no way of knowing if the treatment recommendations that directly follow a positive HIV result are appropriate, *even if HIV were the cause of AIDS*. This fact alone should ring alarm bells regarding medicating pregnant mothers with toxic antiviral drugs. Most people are aware that pregnant women are encouraged to avoid any potentially toxic substance, including caffeine, alcohol, painkillers, and some antibiotics. The lessons of the Thalidomide disaster ought to have been well learned, but apparently the risk of giving birth to a child carrying HIV antibodies is greater than that of any deformity, cancer, or even stillbirth.

Current treatment protocol for pregnant women diagnosed HIV-positive is to administer a course of AZT or some other combination of anti-HIV drugs from the second trimester of pregnancy through delivery, which must be by Cesarean section, as vaginal delivery is considered too risky. The baby is then tested for HIV antibodies and given AZT as well. Often babies who test HIV-positive are simply harboring what are called ghost antibodies inherited from the mother. In the case of such ghost antibodies, they will disappear within nine to eighteen months of birth *in the absence of antiretroviral medication*. It is estimated that more than half of HIV-positive babies revert to negative. The wisdom of providing toxic drugs to these children is highly debatable no matter one's position on HIV and AIDS.

AZT is by no means the only drug available to treat HIV, but it is certainly one of the most toxic, and its symptoms include wasting, anemia, bone marrow suppression, and fulminating white-blood-cell death, making disease from AZT virtually indistinguishable from AIDS itself. What is particularly significant about AZT is that it is among the most common of the drugs approved to prevent mother-to-child transmission of HIV in the US. In other countries, nevirapine has been approved in single-dose use, presumably for administration during labor, but it has not been approved for this purpose in the US, and its use has been implicated in the high-profile death of at least one mother, Joyce Ann Hafford, who died from nevirapine toxicity within days of giving birth.[63]

The treatment of HIV-positive expectant mothers and children remains a matter of much debate, although media reports seem to insist that any fears about mutagenic or teratogenic effects must be quelled in the face of the far greater threat of delivering an HIV-positive child, or having a child die of AIDS.

The question is: what is an AIDS death in a child? Certainly children can die of *Pneumocystis carinii* pneumonia (PCP), or of candidiasis, or any of the other traditional AIDS-defining diseases (though Kaposi's sarcoma is mysteriously absent in children with AIDS as it is in all non-homosexual risk groups). However, one disease that has been added to the AIDS definition, only for children, is "recurrent bacterial infections."[42]

No number is given for what constitutes "recurrent." Putting aside for the moment that many children suffer from recurrent bacterial infections, a more disturbing question arises. Why is this condition *not* AIDS-defining for adults? The traditional definition of an immune deficiency is the inability to fight a multitude of common bacterial infections, but this is absent in AIDS patients. The diseases that AIDS patients succumb to are commonly fungal infections such as *Pneumocystis* and *Candida*, not multiple bacterial infections at all, leading one to question whether AIDS is truly an immune deficiency in the *traditional* sense.

The chief reasons it was initially believed that AIDS is a standard immune deficiency are twofold: patients were getting sick with diseases that were previously rare in "healthy" individuals, and these patients, when tested, showed a significant depletion in the CD4+ subset of the T-cells of their immune system. A decline in CD4+ cells was purported to be the hallmark of the disease and a general barometer of the overall health of the immune system. It was for this reason that scientists focused on searching for a pathogen that was capable of infecting and damaging these very cells.

But what was also known from the beginnings of AIDS— though bizarrely, not investigated to nearly the extent that CD4+ T-cells have been investigated—was that AIDS patients suffered disruption in many subsets of their blood cells. Virtually all of these patients had elevated levels of many different types of antibodies, indicating that something had gone wrong with the "antibody arm" of the immune system. (The existence of such an unusually high level of antibodies, by the way, has been suggested as a serious confounding factor in the alleged specificity of the HIV antibody tests, and this topic will be discussed further in a later chapter.)

Significant understanding as to why AIDS patients, and to a lesser extent, a nontrivial proportion of HIV-positives, experienced highly nontraditional immune deficiencies became possible in the late 1980s, when the subset of CD4+ ("helper") T-cells was further differentiated into two subtypes, Th1 and Th2.[64] The Th1 subset controls what is referred to as "cell-mediated" immunity, and is directed toward *intracellular* pathogens, such as fungi and yeasts. A depletion in the Th1 subset results in the types of opportunistic infections seen in AIDS patients. The Th2 subset is associated with antibody production and "humoral" immunity, and as such effectively directs against mainly bacterial infections. Typically seen in AIDS patients is a reduction in the Th1 subset and an increase in the Th2 subset, leading to a preponderance of opportunistic infections but very few, if any, bacterial infections. Also, an excess in the Th2 subset inevitably leads to excessive antibody production.[64]

Further support for what is called the Th1/Th2 switch can be found by considering where the different subset of T-cells "live."

Th1 cells are primarily found in the bloodstream, whereas Th2 cells remain in the bone marrow and the lymph nodes. Finding a low T-cell count in the bloodstream, therefore, may not mean that any depletion at all has occurred in the *total* CD4+ cell population, but rather that levels of Th1 cells are lowered and those of Th2 cells elevated. Indeed, this explains perfectly the observation that traditional bacterial immune deficiency diseases are typically not seen in AIDS patients.

Another curiosity is the fact that markers for HIV expression have only been found among the Th2 cell types, and not among Th1 cells.[65] This presents a question whose answer should be very interesting indeed: Why does HIV apparently only infect cells whose growth actually *increases* following infection?

It is currently popular to speak not of "AIDS" but of "HIV disease," a final linguistic alteration that cements the circularly derived correlation. But there are more sinister forces at work here. The use of the term "HIV disease" is an effective way of obscuring the fact that "AIDS" today is as ephemeral and difficult to isolate as the retrovirus itself. In the early 1980s, AIDS consisted of only five diseases, Kaposi's sarcoma (KS), *Pneumocystis carinii* pneumonia (PCP), candidiasis, cytomegalovirus, and "gay bowel syndrome." There was also a state referred to as pre-AIDS or "AIDS-related complex," consisting of various systemic abnormalities including weight loss and persistent lymphadenopathy (swelling of the lymph nodes). Despite the fact that KS and PCP have absolutely nothing in common other than being linked by their appearance in a particular segment of society, at least AIDS had a somewhat consistent clinical presentation.

Not only has any specific clinical presentation for AIDS become impossible thanks to the list of twenty-five to thirty, depending on where one lives, AIDS-defining conditions, many of which have absolutely nothing to do with one another or with immune deficiency at all, but the existence of a particular clinical picture that we can call "AIDS" has become confounded by a number of factors.

First, patients are living longer than ever expected. There are people alive and well today who were diagnosed not only HIV-positive but also as having had AIDS itself back in 1984. Popular consensus would say that the increased life expectancy is completely attributable to the antiviral drugs. This is negated by the fact that many of those so diagnosed have either not been taking antiviral drugs, or have taken them very briefly. There is another item to consider, however, and that is the fact that dosages of drugs given today are far lower than in the days of AZT monotherapy. Consequently, people who would never have developed AIDS in the first place—if they had not been coerced into starting antiviral therapy—are simply developing illnesses more slowly than they would have under AZT monotherapy or aggressive HAART.

AIDS is looking less and less like a disease or even a syndrome at all, as all uncomfortable contradictions are swept under the rug, and "HIV disease" has become a name for some combination of the results of three blood tests—antibody, CD4+, and viral load—often in the presence of no disease at all.

CHAPTER 5

Problems with the HIV Tests

By now, many members of my generation, including me, have had an "AIDS test." But what exactly is an "AIDS test"? We already know AIDS isn't a disease, so what are we testing for?

The easy answer is: antibodies to HIV. Everyone knows that. A positive result indicates you were exposed to HIV at one time, developed antibodies to it, and surely the virus is hiding in your body somewhere—because everyone knows that HIV antibodies are *not* protective, quite the opposite: they are a sure sign of imminent death and doom. Brave new viruses follow brave new rules, evidently.*

---

* It has been pointed out that there are a variety of other viruses, most notably herpes simplex, varicella zoster virus (which causes chickenpox but also

(Continued on next page)

It may come as a surprise that no HIV antibody test has been approved by the FDA to diagnose HIV infection *on its own*. Each test must be tested against or used in combination with another unvalidated test, and depending on where you live, it takes a magic combination ranging from three, two, one, or no positive result(s) on three, two, or one unvalidated test(s) to be "confirmed" HIV-positive.

It is also relevant to note that the HIV antibody tests were *never* originally intended as diagnostic tools, but rather as screening tests to guarantee the safety of the blood supply.

The implications of this are so far-reaching as to be, to my mind, absolutely scandalous. Even if we throw away the causation issue, even if we assume for the sake of argument that HIV absolutely does cause AIDS, the fact remains that the HIV antibody tests have been used as a weapon of discrimination ever since testing began. I can think of no medical test that is used the way the HIV antibody test is used.

Ignoring the fact that no medical test should be used to discriminate against anyone, ever, this situation becomes far worse when one considers that the tests being used in this way are some of the worst tests ever manufactured in terms of standardization, specificity, and reproducibility.

---

shingles), and others, that can induce disease long after the establishment of antiviral immunity as evidenced by the appearance of antibodies. Such diseases are often used as arguments for HIV's apparent pathogenicity long after antibody production. What the HIV promoters consistently fail to mention is that in all other cases, the antibody response is weakened and the virus is highly active, meaning that the symptomatic infection appeared thanks to a temporary decline in immunity that allowed for the appearance of the cold sores, the shingles rash, or what have you. HIV, in contrast, is not highly active at any point during final AIDS stages, so the comparison is not apt.

Media advertisements—particularly on music video channels such as MTV, VH1, and BET, popular among preteens, teens, and young adults—have long advocated the concept that "everyone is at risk," and that we should *all* get an HIV test. We've probably all heard the slogan "knowing is beautiful," which leads to the question: Knowing what, exactly?

The push for mass HIV testing appears to be reaching a fever pitch lately, possibly due to the fact that the general public seems to sense that we are *not* all at risk—a conception that AIDS advocates, for reasons which may be entirely altruistic but which are equally likely to be sinister or at best self-serving, believe needs to be changed. A recent campaign by the shoe manufacturer Aldo featured well-known entertainers such as Christina Aguilera and Charlize Theron urging "AIDS awareness and testing"—as though we are not already aware of AIDS, after twenty years of mass media campaigns. Furthermore, the shoe designer Kenneth Cole, recently designated chairman of the board of the American Foundation for AIDS Research (AmFAR), has launched a campaign recently that states, bluntly and absurdly, "We all have AIDS."

With such alarm bells being sounded throughout the mainstream media, it is no wonder that at this time, nearly half of all adults have had at least one HIV test.[17] This test is accompanied by significant anxiety on the part of the person submitting to it, made worse by the fact that one has to wait on tenterhooks for the results to come back, sometimes as long as two weeks. It might seem reasonable for a person to be curious about what, exactly, the test is actually testing *for*, given the stigma associated with a positive result (or even with the fact that one "had to" get tested) and the supposed death sentence associated with this result.

It might seem reasonable to be curious—and it is curious indeed that most people never ask the question.

We assume, based on what we've been told for years by television, newspapers, politicians, and celebrity activists, that this test is measuring the presence or absence of a virus that will eventually kill you in a very nasty manner indeed. No wonder the testing campaign at times seems like a campaign of terror.

When you look at the medical literature and at the documentation provided by the test manufacturers themselves, though, you find out something quite different than what you had first imagined.

Even more shocking than the disclaimers placed in test kits asserting their lack of validation and *lack of FDA approval to diagnose HIV infection* is that patient serum (blood) must be diluted by a factor of fifty to four hundred times before it is tested for HIV antibodies.[8,66]

The two major test kits routinely used for HIV diagnosis are the enzyme-linked immunosorbent assay (ELISA) test and the Western Blot (WB) test. The ELISA is run first, as a "screening" tool, and was first developed on the basis that it would be helpful in screening donated blood for HIV antibodies. Depending on where you live, if your first ELISA is reactive (what we call "positive," a label we shall soon see is quite misleading), you may get a second ELISA. If this ELISA is also reactive, you are tested with a different test, the WB. This is the final "confirmatory" test for HIV infection. It is extremely important to realize that these tests are *all* antibody tests, and they are all used to detect the presence or absence of certain "HIV-specific" antibodies.

Why is this so important? Remember, we're testing for antibodies here. In most cases, antibody tests are used to determine *prior* infection, because the pathogen itself is long gone. In certain cases, such as herpes and syphilis, there is concern about latent infections possibly becoming reactivated some time after the production of antibodies,[†] and so an antibody test is a reasonable measure to take. Antibody tests are done in general because they are cheaper and easier to do than to directly test for viruses or bacteria. However, in all these cases, the antibody tests have been rigorously verified against the gold standard of microbial isolation—that is, the microbe was isolated in pure form and determined to consistently and specifically generate exactly those antibodies being tested for.

Of course, antibody tests all have a certain degree of nonspecificity due to the fact that certain proteins do cross-react. Some false positives occur with all antibody tests, but the rate of false positives for HIV is a particularly outrageous example of this phenomenon. Most of this is no doubt due to the fact that the tests are not verified against viral isolation, but part of the fault lies with the fact that the proteins contained in the test kit are not specific to HIV.

The reason that HIV tests can never be used to diagnose true infection with an exogenous retrovirus is the same reason there is a reasonable correlation between testing HIV-positive and the risk of developing AIDS (and this risk is magnified in the high-prevalence groups). In the early days of AIDS, when the antibody tests were being developed, it was not possible to actually isolate HIV particles and prove the presence of these particles in people diagnosed antibody-positive as well as their absence in those

---

[†]   Notice though that the presence of all such antibodies to latent infection merely indicate the *possibility* that the infection may later reactivate, not the certainty that it will. But with HIV, for some reason as yet never demonstrated in the literature, the presence of antibodies is taken to mean that the infection will not only later reactivate (since it is supposedly never inactive despite its activity being notoriously difficult to observe), but that it will do so in a particularly spectacular fashion, in every single case.

antibody-negative. Instead, cell cultures from AIDS patients were activated using powerful chemicals called mitogens and after this activation, about thirty proteins were found in this mixture, all of which gathered at a density characteristic of retroviruses. A subset of these were specifically attributed to HIV and nothing else, and ten of these are used to define reactivity on the ELISA and Western Blot antibody tests.

The stunning part of this story is how, out of thirty or so possible retroviral proteins, those ten were selected as being specifically from HIV and nothing else. Remember, HIV had not been properly isolated at this point and there was no way of knowing directly that any of these proteins was specific to HIV. So, in an amazing display of circular logic, they simply selected the proteins that most commonly reacted in blood samples of AIDS and pre-AIDS patients.[67,68] No wonder there is a correlation between being HIV-positive and developing AIDS in some risk groups.

Although this reasoning is absolutely scandalous, the problems with the HIV tests do not stop there. The initial ELISA test must be run on serum that has been diluted four hundredfold with a special diluting agent provided by the test manufacturer. This seems rather strange, particularly considering that most antibody tests—for example, the test for antibodies to hepatitis B—are run on undiluted serum, and even those that are diluted are diluted by a very low factor, such as for Epstein-Barr virus, which is diluted tenfold. The only antibody test that has a dilution factor that could possibly be described as approaching that of the HIV ELISA is the rheumatoid factor (RF) antibody test, which must be diluted fortyfold—which is still an order of magnitude lower than the dilution required for the HIV ELISA. (The HIV WB is run at a dilution factor of 50:1.)

One wonders what would happen if the HIV ELISA were run undiluted. Amazingly, there is an answer to this question available. Dr. Roberto Giraldo, a medical doctor working at the Cornell University hospital, ran an experiment in which he tested over one hundred *undiluted* patient samples, including a sample of his own blood, all of which reacted "negative" on ELISA as it is run according to normal testing protocol. He discovered that *every sample reacted* on ELISA when undiluted. This means that 100 percent of samples tested "positive" when undiluted.[8]

While this example alone should be enough to cast significant doubt as to what it is, exactly, that these tests actually detect, it gets worse.

The HIV antibody tests contain a mixture of ten or eleven "HIV-specific" proteins. In the ELISA, the proteins are present as a mixture, and the serum reacts with the proteins in such a way as to cause a color change. The color change is not discrete—meaning that everyone has varying degrees of reaction. It isn't as if those who are really "HIV infected" have the reaction, whereas those who are not show no difference. There are varying degrees of the color change, and a cutoff value has been established, above which the sample is considered reactive or "positive," and below which it is considered negative.

Clearly, this language is absurd, since *positive* and *negative* are polarities and not positions on a sliding scale. Moreover, the decision as to where the cutoff is placed is not universal but is determined by the testing venue and depends on what the test is intended for.[69,70] This is patently ridiculous—like deciding that in Texas "cold" will be 32 degrees but in New Hampshire it will be 25 degrees. Hence, I strenuously object to the terms "positive" and "negative" in the context of HIV tests, since clearly these words are not well defined. "Reactive" and "nonreactive," though still not perfect descriptors of what is actually happening, are more realistic.

With the WB, the proteins are separated out according to their molecular weight in kilodaltons and are then presented as "bands" on a thin nitrocellulose strip, so that a reactive test is determined by a particular combination of reactive protein bands. As with the ELISA, a "positive" results on the WB is not consistently defined. Depending upon the lab or the country in which the lab is located, different combinations of two, three, or four bands are sufficient to diagnose HIV infection.[69]

There is an important question here waiting to be asked: If all these proteins are specific to HIV, shouldn't only one protein be sufficient to diagnose infection? On the other hand, if a person is truly infected, shouldn't their serum react to all ten bands, not just two or three or four?

It turns out that there is ample evidence in the medical literature that cross-reactivity with several of these proteins is *extremely* common in the general, low-risk population. It has been found that between 20 and 40 percent of blood donors from the general population show "indeterminate" WB results, meaning that they have one or two reactive bands, or some combination that "does not fit the criteria for positivity."[60] This means, if the HIV tests are accurate, that these people have antibodies to one or two HIV proteins. (However, in Africa two reactive bands are enough to diagnose infection, and in most places in the US, Canada, and the UK, three bands suffice. The most stringent criteria of four reactive bands—but not the same four—is adhered to by only two countries, France and Australia.)

An extremely comprehensive review of the Western Blot test was published in the journal *Bio/Technology* (now *Nature Bio/ Technology*).[69] It was shown that of the proteins present in the

Western Blot HIV antibody test, the following nonspecificities can be noted:

The protein gp120, which is considered to be a component of the envelope of HIV, and as such being part of the "knobs" or "spikes" on its surface, which enable it to enter an uninfected cell, is not specific to HIV. The proteins gp41, p80, and gp160, are all associated. Specifically, p80, gp120 and gp160 are all considered to be "oligomers" of gp41—which basically means they consist of the appropriate number of gp41 proteins hooked together; gp41, itself, has been shown to be nonspecific and is considered to be a component of cellular actin, ubiquitous in human cells and certainly not specific to HIV.[71,72]

The p24 protein is considered to be synonymous with HIV infection. In fact, newborns are often tested for p24 antigen as a surrogate marker for HIV infection, since antibody tests cannot be used due to the presence of "ghost" antibodies inherited from the mother that persist for up to eighteen months. However, p24 is frighteningly common among individuals at no risk of HIV infection. Serum from blood donors that is nonreactive on ELISA has a 20 to 40 percent chance of being "WB indeterminate," and p24 is the most commonly cross-reacting protein, appearing in 70 percent of indeterminate cases. Furthermore, 41 percent of multiple sclerosis patients who are not ELISA-reactive test positive for p24 antigen. Even more puzzling is that p24 is detected in nowhere near 100 percent of AIDS patients.

In other words, of ELISA-negative serum, 14 to 28 percent tested will have non-HIV-specific reactions to p24. Further, considering that not all AIDS patients have detectable p24, this means the presence of p24 is neither necessary nor sufficient to diagnose HIV infection.

The p18 protein is the second most frequently detected protein in blood donors at no or very low risk of HIV infection. Along with the HIV *pol* protein p32, it has been detected in many situations in which HIV infection is extremely unlikely, and thus cannot be considered to be indicative of HIV infection.

It is germane to note at this point that in all labs, criteria for positivity of the Western Blot test consists of some combination of the above-mentioned proteins—gp160, gp120, gp41, p24, p18, and p32. However, since none of these proteins is specific to HIV, this would be like saying that since dogs have four legs, are furry, wag their tails, and enjoy eating steak, that *any* entity that is furry and enjoys steak must be a dog.

Of course, antibody tests must satisfy three criteria: they must be specific (meaning very few people truly "negative" would test positive), sensitive (meaning very few people truly "positive" would test negative), and they must be precise, or reproducible. The issues of specificity and standardization have been addressed, and following one further comment regarding the specificity of the HIV antibody tests, we shall discuss their lack of precision.

Test manufacturers and AIDS educators commonly claim sensitivity and specificity levels for the HIV antibody tests of 99 percent or better. While this sounds like an impressive figure, it is meaningless in light of the fact that the aforementioned sensitivity and specificity are estimated by comparing antibody tests against one another and not against HIV itself. However, the problems are considerably worse than this.

Suppose for the sake of argument that these values reflect the true accuracy of the HIV test. HIV is thought to be present in about 0.4 percent of the US population, or in about one of 250 randomly selected Americans. Suppose that we were to administer an HIV test to ten thousand randomly selected Americans. In such a random sample, we would expect about forty "true positives," with the remainder, or 9960 people being negative. A 99 percent sensitivity would mean that 1 percent of those truly positive would actually test negative. With forty people positive, *perhaps* one person would register false negative. So it appears that the test is really quite acceptable as far as eliminating false negatives is concerned.

However, a 99 percent specificity level means that 1 percent of those truly negative would test positive; 1 percent of 9960 is approximately one hundred people, so we can see that the number of false positives would outnumber the true positives by a factor of one hundred to forty, or 2.5! This is because the prevalence of HIV in the population is so low. As the prevalence increases, we get fewer false positives. This factor of true positives to total positives is know as the positive predictive value (PPV) of the test, and it indicates what percentage of all positives we can expect to be true positives. A PPV of 40/140 means that in the total population, *we can expect only about 35 percent of all positive tests to be "true" positives.*

If we test outside the risk groups, the prevalence of HIV goes down to about one in five thousand, or 0.02 percent. Testing ten thousand non-risk group Americans would yield *two* true positives. However, we would obtain approximately one hundred false positives in this case, and the PPV is less than 2 percent! Clearly, testing outside the risk groups would mean that almost everyone who would test positive would be a false positive, and, extrapolating to the general population, tens of thousands of people would be terrorized and put on poisonous drugs for no reason—a medical disaster.

Repeat testing would eliminate many of these false positives, but not all of them, as we will see. Perhaps the most striking example of the imprecision, or nonreproducibility, of the WB test, can be found in the Army study by Colonel Burke and coauthors. In all, 135,187 military applicants at very low risk for HIV infection were selected and tested using the protocol of an initial screening ELISA, followed by a second ELISA if the first was reactive, then a WB if the second ELISA was also reactive, and finally a second WB if the first WB was also positive.[73] They found that on initial ELISA screening, six thousand individuals tested positive. Upon repeating the ELISA, two thousand people were negative, leaving only four thousand positive specimens. These four thousand specimens were then tested. Among those whose first WB was reactive, eighty had a positive WB followed by a negative repeat WB. In the clinical setting, the testing would have stopped at the first positive WB, leaving eighty people determined to be truly negative in the Army study who would have been given a death sentence if they were tested by their doctors. How many, if all Americans were tested as per the CDC's recommendations, would be given a death sentence *even with repeat testing?* Since eighty of 135,187 false positives would not have been eliminated by accepted test procedures, this means *more than 170,000 Americans would be given a death sentence for no reason.*

The problem is further confounded in the ELISA test, since the proteins are present as a mixture, and there is no way of knowing what sort of cross-reactivity may be occurring. It certainly seems as though virtually every human would have a reactive ELISA if the test were run undiluted, so what does this mean about the specificity of the test? There is no other interpretation than to say that the test is a nonspecific test, like the test for RF antibodies. If the tests were highly specific (which is doubtful), the only possible explanation would be that more or less everyone has been exposed to HIV at some time, but some people simply produce more antibodies than others, and these people's antibodies still react even under a four hundred fold dilution.

Assuming that this explanation is not reasonable, which I suspect to be the case, the other possible reason for the results indicated above is that the tests are simply nonspecific and cannot in any way diagnose infection with a *particular* microbe. The best they can do is to detect a condition called *hypergammaglobulinemia*, meaning having too many antibodies to too many things. This explanation is perfectly consistent with the finding of reactive specimens in most AIDS patients. It has been known since the beginning of the AIDS epidemic that AIDS patients had generally been exposed to a vast number of infections (and occasionally, recreational drugs) prior to testing positive. Since infections, as well as drug use, induce antibodies, it is no surprise that the likelihood of cross-reactions will increase. It is also known that having so many antibodies indicates a problem with the antibody arm of the immune system, and that having such problems typically accompanies a deficiency in cell-mediated immunity—exactly what is observed in AIDS patients.

It is relevant to note that about 40 percent of the human genome is composed of what are called *RNA transposable elements*.[74] RNA is composed of a single strand of nucleotides (rather than the familiar double helix of DNA) and replicates differently than does DNA. The word *transposable* means that they can move or "jump" around, as well as cleave and form *endogenous retroviruses*. Endogenous retroviruses are the same in structure as "conventional" exogenous retroviruses, as HIV is purported to be, having at least three genes, *gag*, *pol*, and *env*. This is significant because, among other reasons, it is impossible to distinguish an endogenous retrovirus from an exogenous retrovirus simply by looking at a picture. This is part of what makes retroviruses so different from "ordinary" viruses.

Human beings are full of retroviruses that start out as retroviral sequences in the genome. They are expressed an endogenous retroviruses whenever cells are decaying at a higher rate than normal and often when cells are dividing and growing at a higher rate than normal. This is a major confounding factor for the HIV tests, because during times of disease or growth, such as pregnancy, a higher than normal level of endogenous retroviruses will be expressed, and we form antibodies to their proteins. This greatly increases the chances of cross-reactivity, and it at least partly explains why people whose health is compromised in the first place are more likely to test HIV-positive, as well as why people who test HIV-positive are more likely to become ill. The retroviruses are simply a marker for cell decay and/or division.

Furthermore, some of the known human endogenous retroviruses (for instance, HERV-K and HERV-W) not only produce antibodies that cross-react with the HIV test,[75] but they have RNA sequences that are very similar to those of HIV, and these sequences are very likely to be mistaken by the viral load PCR as fragments belonging to HIV. (Viral load PCR does not measure intact viruses but rather fragments believed to belong to HIV, as we will discuss further later in this chapter.)

Endogenous retroviruses are primarily transmitted perinatally, from mother to child. Perinatal transmission is presumed to be the most efficient mode of HIV transmission, which should raise suspicions as to whether there is sufficient information to conclude that HIV is even exogenous at all, particularly given the lack of solid evidence of sexual or perenteral (blood-to-blood via infected needles) transmission.[76–79]

The idea that HIV tests might be a nonspecific marker for an immune system with a broken antibody arm is further strengthened by the fact that these tests have never been validated against the gold standard of HIV isolation. Since the diagnosis HIV-positive carries with it such a stigma and the potential for outrageous denial of human rights, it is only humane that doctors, AIDS researchers, and test manufacturers would want to make absolutely certain that the tests they are promoting are completely verifiable in the best possible way.

This is not happening. These tests have never been verified against the presence of HIV because, to date, there is no clear evidence that HIV has been isolated in such a manner as to be acceptable as a gold standard for antibody tests. By isolation, HIV researchers usually mean successful culturing, which merely means that certain chemical reactions indicating phenomena consistent with HIV have been observed.

Etienne de Harven published a paper in 1998 that was highly critical of the methods used for isolating HIV and the other human retroviruses, as well as the subsequent development of the antibody tests.

When, around 1980, Gallo and his followers attempted to demonstrate that certain retroviruses [can cause disease in humans], to the best of my bibliographical recollection, electron microscopy was never used to demonstrate directly viremia (the presence of virus in the blood) in the studied patients. Why? Most probably electron-micrographic results were negative, and swiftly ignored! But over-enthusiastic retrovirologists continued to rely on the identification of so-called "viral markers" attempting to salvage their hypothesis . . . ELISA, then Western Blot tests were hastily developed, at sizable profits eagerly split between the Pasteur Institute and the US. "Seropositivity" (based on these two tests) became synonymous with the disease, itself, plunging an entire generation into behavioral panic, and exposing thousands of people to "preventative" AZT therapy which actually hastened the appearance of severe or lethal immunodeficiency syndrome.[30]

HIV researchers will swear up and down that HIV has been properly isolated and that such apparently sensible criteria as separation of viral particles from everything else and proof of their existence as shown by clear electron micrographs are not necessary.[‡] You might think that with the hundreds of billions of dollars spent so far on HIV, there would have been by now a successful attempt to demonstrate HIV isolation by publication of proper electron micrographs. The fact that there has not indicates quite strongly that no one has been able to do it. Since the "isolation problem" has long been an argument put forth by scientists questioning HIV, it seems that if it were possible to resolve this problem, mainstream researchers would be eager to do it if only to shut such dissenters up.

While this may be alarming enough in and of itself, it is of particular concern when one considers that every day people are given a diagnosis of imminent death based on a test whose value as a diagnostic tool is very dubious indeed. One need only consider some of the disclaimers included in any of the popular test kits:

ELISA testing alone cannot be used to diagnose AIDS.
                    —*Abbott Laboratories test kit (Abbott 1997)*

Do not use this kit as the sole basis for determining HIV infection.
                    —*Epitope Western Blot kit (Epitope 1997)*

---

‡   Of course, there are a very few viruses that can only be cultured. However, these examples contain ample further evidence of pathogenicity.

The amplicor HIV-1 monitor test is not intended to be used as a screening test for HIV, nor a diagnostic test to confirm the presence of HIV infection.

—*Roche viral load kit (Roche 1996)*

As to so-called viral load, most people are not aware that tests for viral load are neither approved nor recommended by the FDA to diagnose HIV infection. This is why an "AIDS test" is still an anti-body test. Viral load, however, *is* used to estimate the health status of those already diagnosed HIV-positive. But there are very good reasons to believe it does not work at all. Viral load uses either polymerase chain reaction (PCR) or a technique called branched-chain DNA amplification (bDNA). PCR is the same technique used for "DNA fingerprinting" at crime scenes where only trace amounts of materials can be found. PCR essentially mass-produces DNA and RNA so that it can be seen. If something has to be mass-produced to even be seen, and the result of that mass pro-duction is used to estimate how much of a pathogen there is, it might lead a person to wonder how relevant the pathogen was in the first place. Specifically, how could something so hard to find, even using the most sensitive and sophisticated technology, completely decimate the immune system? While not magnifying anything directly, bDNA nevertheless only looks for fragments of DNA believed, but not proven, to be components of the genome of HIV—but there is no evidence to say that these fragments exist in other genetic sequences unrelated to HIV or to any virus.

While at first glance it might seem completely reasonable to estimate the quantity of a pathogen by amplifying it and then using the amplification formula to back-calculate for the true quantity, there are serious problems with this approach. As Mark Craddock explains, the efficiency of PCR must be *perfect* in order to obtain an accurate value.[31] This is rarely the case. If the efficiency is off by even a small amount, the error has the potential to increase (or decrease) exponentially because PCR amplifies up to forty-five times. Even the mainstream literature[36] admits that viral load testing overestimates infectious virus by a factor of at least sixty thousand. This means that a viral load of sixty thousand corresponds to at most one infectious viral particle. In the aforementioned Piatak paper, fully one-half of their patients with detectable viral loads had no evidence of virus by culture.

More damning evidence against the use of viral load as an indicator of clinical health is given by Mark Craddock in his rebuttal to the Durban Declaration. In his letter, which remains unpublished to this day,§ he examined the patients in the Piatak paper. Using their CD4+ T-cell counts, viral loads, and measurements of virus by culture, he computed correlation coefficients on all pairwise combinations. A correlation coefficient is a numerical value that measures the strength of the relationship between two variables. A correlation coefficient close to 1 means a nearly 100 percent association, whereas a correlation coefficient near 0 means there is no association. Statisticians generally view any correlation coefficient less than 0.5 as indicating very poor correlation.

Craddock's computations revealed that among all pairwise combinations, the correlation coefficients were close to zero. This is extremely relevant, because it means that T-cell count has no effect on viral load, viral load has no relation to infectious virus levels, and infectious viral levels have nothing to do with T-cell count. In other words, *all laboratory tests used to assess the severity of HIV infection are virtually worthless.*

---

§   see http://healtoronto.com/durban/craddock.html.

It is worth noting at this point that viral load, like antibody tests, has never been verified against the gold standard of HIV isolation—bDNA uses PCR as a gold standard, PCR uses antibody tests as a gold standard, and antibody tests use each other. None use HIV itself.[80]

It is also germane to note that Kary Mullis, the *inventor* of the PCR technique, which is the primary tool used in assessing viral load, wastes no opportunity to publicly decry the misuse of PCR to quantify viral load. Dr. Mullis has called the HIV/AIDS hypothesis "one hell of a mistake: and has stated that "quantitative PCR is an oxymoron."[81]

However, I would argue that the real problem with the administration of HIV antibody tests lies not with the tests themselves but with how they are essentially used as weapons of terror. This medical terrorism reached new heights in June 2006 with the CDC's new HIV testing guidelines, which recommend that everyone between the ages of thirteen and sixty-five be tested for antibodies to HIV. Prior to the publication of these guidelines, HIV tests were not standard practice, due partly to the fact that pre- and post-test counseling was to be given alongside the tests, making the testing process expensive and time consuming. In general, to get an HIV test, one either had to visit an STD or HIV clinic and request to be tested, or one needed to specifically ask one's doctor. (Other portions of the population, such as blood donors, military recruits, and patients undergoing certain hospital procedures, are subject to mandatory testing, but these segments of society do not comprise a large proportion of the population.)

Hence, it is not surprising that the vast majority of HIV tests have traditionally been sought by individuals in risk groups or people who had some good reason to believe they had contracted HIV. The new testing guidelines could change all this, and as a result, the number of false positives will soar. This is owing to Bayes' Law, which states that the higher the prevalence of a pathogen in the population, the higher will be the positive predictive value (PPV) of the test—that is, the lower the rate of false positives will be. The problem, as we have seen, is that in a population with low prevalence, the PPV will plummet and the rate of false positives will soar. Of course, many of these false positives can be eliminated by repeat testing, but as the Army study noted above clearly demonstrates, repeat testing will not eliminate all of these false positives.

Why is this a problem? Aside from the fact that many people who are perfectly healthy will be coerced into undergoing a regimen of medication that will inevitably cause long term toxic effects (and often death), a more sinister complication is the violation in human rights that occurs following a positive HIV test. Every state in the US and every province in Canada maintains a list of "HIV carriers" in that region. Once diagnosed HIV-positive, medical and life insurance can be denied, some careers may be terminated, but worst of all, a death sentence is given and, contrary to every other disease known to man, even cancers that are generally 100 percent fatal, hope is not allowed. Women are encouraged to abort their babies, and if they choose to carry their pregnancy to term, in many states they are forced to take antiretroviral drugs, and these drugs are forced on their babies as well. The babies must be born by Cesarean section, and in many states the highly beneficial practice of breastfeeding is illegal.

Clearly, the "HIV test" needs to be thoroughly reappraised as a diagnostic tool. Results of this test should not be used to discriminate against anyone, especially since the test itself is so unreliable. But more urgently, *at the very least,* the HIV antibody tests ought to be rigorously verified against the actual presence of HIV itself. This has never been done.

CHAPTER 6

Why There Is No Evidence
That HIV Causes AIDS

The astounding lack of evidence supporting the HIV paradigm can be summarized in both biological and epidemiological terms. For the sake of simplicity, I will present a summary of the major biological criticisms first and will follow with the epidemiological inconsistencies. Also, please notice that there is considerable overlap between this chapter and the previous one, since many of the reasons to doubt the validity of the HIV tests also cast doubt on the ability of HIV to cause any disease.

AIDS is said to be caused by a dramatic loss of the immune system's T-cells, said loss being presumably caused by HIV. However, as recently as March of 2006, longtime HIV researcher Dr. Zvi

Grossman stated, in a paper published in *Nature Medicine* that examined the various hypotheses of HIV-mediated T-cell depletion, and found them all wanting: "The pathogenic and physiologic processes leading to AIDS remain a conundrum."[82]

Why is it that still no one understands the dynamics of the fundamental disease process—that is, how are T-cells actually killed by HIV? Early models assumed that HIV killed T-cells directly, by what is referred to as lysis. An infected cell lyses, or bursts, when the internal viral burden is so high that it can no longer be contained, just like your grocery bag breaks when it's too full. This is the accepted mechanism of pathogenesis for virtually all other pathogenic viruses. But it became clear that HIV did *not* kill T-cells in this manner, and this concept was abandoned, to be replaced by various other ones, each of which resulted in very different models and, therefore, different predictions.[83] Which model was *correct* was never clear.

There is still no consensus as to how HIV kills T-cells, although the notion of apoptosis, also known as programmed cell death, has become popular despite no real evidence of its occurrence. In laboratory experiments where apoptosis has been demonstrated in HIV-infected cell cultures, apoptosis is detected only after the addition of powerful chemical stimulants called mitogens. However, *uninfected* cultures that have been mitogenically stimulated also demonstrate apoptosis.[35] It is claimed that the presence of the envelope protein gp120 and its oligomer, gp41, prime CD4+ T-cells early on for a future process of programmed cell death. However, it is known that neither gp120 nor gp41 are specific to HIV, and gp41 is presumed by Luc Montagnier's group to be cellular actin, a ubiquitous component of all cells. The conundrum of how proteins that are present in normal cells could possibly induce apoptosis only in the cells of "HIV-positive" individuals has never been resolved. Furthermore, such apoptosis-inducing proteins as gp120, tat, and nef are present in other retroviruses including human endogenous retroviruses, yet these retroviruses are not thought to induce apoptosis to anywhere near the extent that HIV supposedly does.

HIV is possibly the most studied microbe in history—certainly it is the best funded—yet there is still no agreed-upon method of pathogenesis. There are good reasons to believe that HIV is not pathogenic at all. One important reason is the fundamental nature of retroviruses themselves.

Retroviruses were popular in the 1970s "War on Cancer" research program as candidates for cancer-causing viruses because, unlike more pathogenic viruses, retroviruses do not kill the cells they infect. In fact, in some instances it was found that the cells infected by retroviruses actually grew at a faster than normal rate. However, despite findings that some retroviruses did seem to be associated with tumors in animals, the quest to find a cancer-causing retrovirus has been a failure.[84]

A retrovirus is nothing more than RNA with an outer protein shell. The shell enables it to bind to cells of the type it infects, and once it gains entry, the outer coating disappears and the RNA is transcribed to DNA and is incorporated *as provirus* into the host cell's own genome. It is for this reason that retroviruses are called enveloped viruses, and it is also the reason that it is very difficult to distinguish between *exogenous* retroviruses (those that originate outside the body from a foreign invader) and *endogenous* retroviruses (those that are manufactured from our own retroviral-like genetic sequences* under conditions of cellular stress, including disease).

---

* It is estimated that 3 percent of the human genome is retroviral in nature. This amount of genetic information is several hundreds of times larger than the genome of HIV.

It should be clear why an enveloped virus would not kill its host cell, as it is completely dependent on the host to replicate. Instead, replication is accomplished by means of new viral particles budding from the host cell's membrane. However, this productivity is low in the case of HIV, as only approximately one in ten thousand 4+ T-cells is ever productively infected,[85] which is why finding actual HIV in humans is extraordinarily difficult. It has been proposed that free HIV is not responsible for the vast majority of cellular infection, and instead that direct cell-to-cell infection is the dominant mode of transmission within the host.

If HIV really does cause the destruction of an extraordinary number of CD4+ T-cells, it would be a most unorthodox virus indeed, as it would have the distinction of being the first retrovirus that caused cell destruction outside of the laboratory. (Note that "a retrovirus" is a subset of a class of "RNA viruses." I have been asked numerous times why it is that RNA viruses such as Ebola and hantavirus can cause disease, but the RNA virus HIV does not. The answer is that these are quite simply *not* the same type of viruses. RNA-containing viruses that are not retroviruses are not enveloped and can indeed induce lysis, killing their host cells in the same way that "traditional" DNA-containing viruses do.)

Another conundrum is the difficulty in culturing active HIV from AIDS patients at all—and this doesn't even consider the real difficulties encountered in properly isolating HIV at all, a feat many researchers argue has never been accomplished. As has been discussed in previous chapters, before the publication of the Ho/ Wei papers in 1995, a major thorn in the side of the HIV hypothesis was that negligible amounts of virus were ever to be found— whether one was sick, well, or dying from AIDS, virus titers (as measured by culturing, which generally involves at best detection of reverse transcription, or of p24, or of retroviral-like particles, none of which is specific to HIV) were so low, at about one viral particle per milliliter or even zero, as to be able to explain HIV's allegedly ferocious pathogenesis.

The farcical concept of viral load was invented to create the illusion of correcting this embarrassing fact. However, as we discussed, viral load does not correlate with infectious viruses and thus, even according to HIV theory, cannot possibly have anything to do with illness. To best illustrate the ridiculous level of illogic some HIV scientists can display when confronted with these conundrums, I refer to the experience that Dr. David Rasnick had at a Gordon Conference on AIDS in 1997, which he attended to present a poster that disputed the hypothesis that anti-HIV drugs stop working because of the high mutation rate of HIV.

> In the discussion period of Mellors' lecture, I decided to return to the questions that I'd wanted Markowitz to answer, about the meaning of "viral load." After all, that was the heart of the matter: Mellors' call to discard clinical endpoints [e.g. to consider only surrogate markers such as viral loads as measures of treatment success, disregarding clinical health] was only as valid as the "viral load" figures with which he wished to replace them.
>
> For starters, I wanted to compare his answers to Markowitz's. So I repeated my question about the relation between "viral load" and infectious doses. Mellors responded by proclaiming, "Viral load has nothing to do with infectivity!"
>
> Ah-ha! Now I had a second HIV big shot admitting that "viral load" figures did not indicate infectious HIV.
>
> Assuming that "viral load" testing accurately counted HIV, and that infectious dose testing accurately counted

infectious HIV, I offered my 99.8 percent figure from the Ho/Markowitz paper as the fraction of circulating HIV that was non-infectious.

Non-infectious HIV, then, is the source of RNA and proteins—including protease—from which the genetics and other characteristics of HIV are derived.

He agreed. (How could he not?)

Now I had him. Since non-infectious viruses have no conceivable clinical relevancy, then neither could any of the data derived from them.

What's the significance of all the non-infectious HIV? I asked. I had no idea how he could work himself out of this corner, but even I was stunned by his response: "The non-infectious particles [HIV] are pathogenic."

Now here was a first. I don't think that anybody's ever gone on record before proposing that non-infectious virus could cause disease.

I sat there flabbergasted, noticing the murmur that had broken out. In my astonished state I realized there was nothing else to be said.

In the meantime, the session was declared over, the time allotted for discussion having been exhausted by my cross-examination, with no one else having had time to pose questions.

My God, I thought. Talk about a rich source of research opportunity. The pathogenicity of non-infectious viruses. Anybody familiar with the antibody response and the premise of vaccinations can appreciate the revolutionary nature (and implausibility) of this idea.

My sense is that the audience did, given the intense murmuring, which continued even after the lecture had been dismissed. On the way out of the room an Indian scientist grabbed my arm and asked, "Did you hear that?"

Indeed I had. AIDS was caused by a deadly army of viral corpses.[86]

More perplexing is the fact that no two identical HIV genomes have ever been obtained *in vivo*—even from the same person.[87] This observation has led some researchers to consider that HIV is a "quasi-species" of virus. Others claim that this genetic diversity is the result of HIV's alleged high mutation rate, unprecedented in the history of viruses. Another disturbing possibility that arises is that much of the genetic material attributed to HIV is in fact DNA or RNA from decaying cells, which are capable of producing retroviral-like particles when stressed or dying in large quantities. Human beings are filled with such *endogenous* retroviruses, which are expressed under conditions of cellular stress and decay. Whether one believes that this stress exacerbates the expression of an exogenous retrovirus HIV, or that it is an endogenous, non-infectious retrovirus, or simply a "viral mirage," this information casts serious doubt on the validity of viral load testing or of using either reverse transcriptase or retroviral-like particles or genetic sequences as markers for HIV.

The epidemiology of HIV and AIDS is puzzling and unclear as well. In spite of the fact that AIDS cases increased rapidly from their initial observation in the early 1980s and reached a peak in 1993 before declining rapidly, the number of HIV-positive individuals in the US has remained virtually constant at one million since the advent of widespread HIV antibody testing, as discussed in the Introduction. Again, this cannot be due to anti-HIV therapy, since the annual mortality rate of North American HIV-positives is much higher, at a value somewhere between 6.7 and 8.8 percent, than would be the approximately 1 to 2 percent global mortality rate of HIV-positives, assuming all AIDS cases were fatal in a given year. This fact, as well as the disparities between HIV and AIDS in men and women, motivated Henry Bauer, emeritus dean of science at Virginia Polytechnic Institute and State University, to perform a comprehensive analysis of the CDC's own data from 1985 to the present say.[6,17,88] What he found was shocking.

In this devastating analysis, Bauer points out that many of the epidemiological aspects of HIV that are utterly incompatible with the hypothesis that it causes AIDS.

For instance, HIV had been present everywhere in the US in every population tested, including repeat blood donors and military recruits, at a virtually constant rate since testing began in 1985. It is deeply confusing that a virus thought to have been brought to the AIDS epicenters of New York City, San Francisco, and Los Angeles in the early 1970s could possibly have spread so rapidly at first, yet have stopped spreading completely as soon as testing began.

But the centerpiece of what he noticed was that positive HIV tests show an astonishing regularity across lines of age, gender, race, and geographic location unlike what one would expect from a sexually transmitted infection. Although there was a correlation between regions with high AIDS incidence and high HIV prevalence, AIDS incidence was nowhere near as strong an indicator for HIV-positivity as were other variables. The strongest correlate was race, with the shocking fact that Black teenagers from places with very low AIDS incidence were more than twice as likely to test HIV-positive as the average non-Black teenager from places of high AIDS incidence.

Bauer shows that according to official CDC data complied from testing facilities such as blood banks, prisons, military and job corps testing sites, hospitals, STD clinics, and more, the frequency of positive HIV tests follows the identical distribution over age and race in every group tested. This includes the lowest-risk groups—repeat blood donors and members of the Marine Corps. In every category, without exception, the frequency of positive HIV tests declines from birth into the teen years, increases steadily into middle age, and then begins to fall. The prevalence is nowhere zero, even among groups presumed to be at no risk of infection.

Furthermore, the HIV prevalence ratio in all groups could be categorized by race as follows: from lowest to highest incidence, HIV occurred in the racial categories Asian,[†] Caucasian, Native American, Hispanic, and Black.

In summary, accumulated data from years of testing indicate that the levels of HIV in the population are unchanging geographically—always higher in the East and the South than in the West and Midwest, unchanging in number, and far too consistent over racial groups to be consistent with the irregularities of AIDS in the population. All the epidemiological evidence to date strongly indicates that whatever testing HIV-positive signifies, it is clearly not a reliable indicator of the risk of ever developing AIDS.

---

†   This belies the reports that one of the reasons Asian countries supposedly have higher rates of HIV and AIDS than the West is that Asians lack the alleged genetic mutation that supposedly protects people from contracting HIV. If this were so, Asians in North America should have higher rates of infection than whites, which is not the case.

CHAPTER 7

Sociological Implications of AIDS

On April 23, 1984, the "probable cause of AIDS" had been identified and was announced to the world via press conference. Robert Gallo, PhD, of the NIH, and Margaret Heckler, secretary of Health and Human Services for the Reagan administration, presented this information, which was then broadcast the world over and reported on extensively in newspapers and magazines for weeks, months, years afterward.

The story of AIDS began long before the fateful 1984 press conference. At least as early as mid-1980, reports began to surface of a small group of gay men who were dying from a strange pneumonia and a hitherto rare—and *not* previously fatal—form of skin cancer called Kaposi's sarcoma. The first five men with AIDS were patients of Michael Gottlieb who used a new technology that enabled technicians to count not just the total number of white blood cells a patient has but the number of each *subset* of T-cells. Using this new technology—which coincidentally came into existence and was patented at the beginning of the AIDS era—Gottlieb was able to determine that these men suffered from an unusually low number of the white blood cell subset known as helper T-cells.

The hunt for an agent capable of selectively targeting and depleting this subset of white blood cells was on. In the early days, all manner of infectious and noninfectious causes was considered, but the dogged determination of the retrovirus hunters encouraged some zealous scientists to consider that the target was probably a retrovirus capable of entering the CD4+ T-cells. Robert Gallo had previously discovered two other human retroviruses, HTLV-I and HTLV-II, that were tropic for CD4+ T-cells, so when he found evidence implicating a new retrovirus in some AIDS patients (temporarily christened HTLV-III and now and forever known to the world as HIV), all questions about causation came to an abrupt halt. At the time, the retrovirus seemed to supply all the answers we needed, and thus began work on a cure and a vaccine that was promised by 1986.

Twenty years after the cure was promised to have arrived, there is none, and there likely never will be a vaccine. A massive industry has been built around T-cell testing, viral load testing, antibody testing, and drug development. Drugs have been developed to lower viral load and drugs have been developed to alleviate the sometimes horrific effects of the primary drugs. An entire plastic surgery industry has been put in place to mask the loss and redistribution of fat caused by the drugs.

What good has come of this? How many peoples' lives have actually been *improved* by an HIV-positive diagnosis? Who is better off from this campaign of psychological terror?

The nails in the coffin of the dead HIV/AIDS paradigm have been hammered long ago, by a long list of scientists and medical researchers. The AIDS orthodoxy's only counters to the points made and the questions raised consist of *ad hominem* attacks including the use of the word "denialist," as well as stating that dissenting views have long since been "discredited," without any reference to exactly *where* these views have been discredited. Unfortunately, words are powerful, and personal attacks are very effective at silencing people. Even a cursory examination of the literature reveals that the "discrediting" of dissenting views takes place entirely within non-peer-reviewed outlets such as the anonymously authored NIH/NIAID document "The Evidence That HIV Causes AIDS," and the Durban Declaration—both of which have been thoroughly refuted.

The persistence of this intellectually bankrupt theory in the public mind is thanks entirely to the campaign of fear, discrimination, and terror that has been waged aggressively by a powerful group of people whose sole motivation was and is behavior control. Yes, the money and the vast interests of the pharmaceutical industry and government-funded scientists are important, but the seeds of the HIV/AIDS hypothesis are sown with fear. If the fear were to end, the myth would end.

To understand the sociological motivations behind the HIV/ AIDS paradigm, one must understand the racism and homophobia that has persisted in society for centuries. It is only very recently in the timeline of history that gays and Blacks have been accorded equal rights under the law—rights that Caucasians and heterosexuals have enjoyed since time immemorial. To understand the racism and homophobia behind the very definition of AIDS, one only needs to consider the official party line: AIDS infected humans when Africans consumed or did strange things with monkeys, and it has been spread throughout the world by gay men and sexually promiscuous, prostitute-visiting Black Africans.

This ridiculous concept is utterly intellectually bankrupt—the evidence for an African origin for HIV, much less AIDS, is slim indeed and is based entirely on the hypothesis that Africans have been doing strange things with monkeys which magically permitted not one but two distinct retroviruses, HIV-1 and HIV-2, to somehow jump to humans and start causing massive immune deficiency the likes of which has never before been caused by a single—let alone two distinct—infectious agent. For this to be true, these two new retroviruses must be pretty new in monkeys, too, since nothing has changed regarding how Africans relate to monkeys in the last forty or so years, and logically, such a zoonotic jump, if it were possible, should have happened long ago. For this to be true, AIDS ought to have existed in Africa *significantly before* it existed in New York City, Los Angeles, and San Francisco, rather than *after* (1983), which is what happened.

Scientists jumped to these conclusions because they did not have any hard evidence. The first five men with AIDS were not sexually involved with one another, so why was a sexually transmitted cause considered to be so likely? And of Gallo's cohort of seventy-two homosexuals with AIDS, only twenty-six had any trace of HIV. Yet somehow HIV (and therefore AIDS) was considered sexually transmittable. This conclusion was arrived at not by the traditional method of proving an infection is indeed an STI, which involves microbial isolation and contact tracing, but rather by simply assuming sexual transmission. Laboratory studies of "HIV," in which researchers do experiments showing things like "HIV" not being able to penetrate latex or "HIV" being able to infect monkeys when rectally injected, do not use HIV particles at all, but rather molecular biology experiments consisting of combinations of proteins that trigger an antibody reaction. So how do we know anything about what HIV really does, where it came from, and even what it is?

The answer is: we don't, anymore than we did back in 1984. Despite the fact that other viruses (cytomegalovirus and herpes virus, to give just two examples) were far more prevalent in AIDS patients than HIV ever was, the HIV train started rolling and hasn't lost momentum since. Would this have happened if the first five AIDS patients had been heterosexuals in the prime of their lives?

Many of the biggest crimes committed by the AIDS orthodoxy are psychosocial and not medical at all. People far more well versed than me have exhaustively exposed the level of iatrogenic harm that has been done to HIV-positive individuals by anti-HIV medications, and these arguments remain relevant to this day.[37,50,89] However, I believe more attention needs to be given to the discrimination leveled against these people, as well as the death-cult mentality surrounding "HIV positivity."

It is absolutely stunning that the notion that HIV= AIDS=DEATH has been so firmly entrenched in the public mindset and has been perpetuated by medical personnel and public health "educators." Virtually every other disease known to man is accompanied by some hope of recovery—not so with AIDS.

From the mail that I have received in response to articles published on Lew Rockwell's website, I can attest to the fact that there are many people living healthy lives twenty years after an HIV diagnosis and, furthermore, that a significant number of people remain healthy fifteen or twenty years after an actual *AIDS* diagnosis, without benefit of anti-HIV drugs. Why then does hope not ring eternal for AIDS patients?

Currently, "HIV disease" is classified into four stages, from asymptomatic to AIDS. "Stage 4 HIV disease" refers to a CD4+

T-cell count of less than two hundred or the presence of opportunistic infections.[42] Remarkably, it is stated in plain language that once an individual has been classified as Stage 4, they can never return to any of the lower stages, even if their CD4+ count rebounds or they recover from illness. This is remarkable and totally unprecedented in the history of medicine. A cancer patient is allowed to recover, but an AIDS patient (whatever that means) can never recover, *by definition*, even if their health returns to normal.

The psychological effects of an HIV diagnosis are profound. Further, the psychological effects of the *fear* of an HIV diagnosis are often made manifest in physical symptoms that mimic AIDS—so much so that the term "AIDS phobia" and "AFRAIDS" were coined to describe a syndrome. This syndrome consists of symptoms such as weight loss, gastrointestinal disturbances, night sweats, and flu-like ailments, and it occurs in people who have recently had close contact with people they suspected might be HIV-positive—*even though the "AFRAIDS" sufferer repeatedly tested negative.*

The discrimination leveled against those given an HIV-positive diagnosis has reached a level not seen since leprosy was common. HIV-positives are the modern equivalent of lepers (and in Cuba, where they are quarantined, are even treated as such), despite the fact that all mainstream evidence reveals the infectivity of HIV, even in intimate contact, to be so negligible as to be incapable of sustaining any sort of epidemic. Although education campaigns commonly claim that "we're all at risk," and "AIDS does not discriminate," most Americans are well aware that people really do believe AIDS does discriminate.

Perhaps the most illustrative example of the twisted way in which HIV is viewed as the perpetrator of all evil is the ongoing story of Christine Maggiore and Eliza Jane Scovill. Christine was diagnosed HIV-positive in 1992 and volunteered for several years as an "AIDS educator" before she began to question the basis for her diagnosis. Eventually, any meaning it might have held for her was gone and she founded Alive and Well AIDS Alternatives, a support group for HIV-positive individuals who did not want to bow to conventional HIV/AIDS theories.

Christine married filmmaker Robin Scovill and gave birth to two healthy children, Charlie and Eliza Jane. Indeed, she and her family have remained so healthy that many proponents of the HIV/AIDS paradigm have put forth the hypothesis that Christine is not really HIV-positive. As Jeanne Bergman said in the *New York Press*:

> False negative tests are extremely rare, while false posi-
> tives are much more common, though infrequent. This
> fact and all the other evidence available strongly suggest
> that Maggiore was never infected by HIV . . . Most people
> would be thrilled to know that they were uninfected, but
> Maggiore was unwilling to give up the spotlight. This HIV
> pretender twisted her good health and the marginal inci-
> dence of false positives into a lucrative* new racket—selling
> HIV denialism and bragging about her good life "without
> pharmaceutical treatments or fear of AIDS." But of course
> Maggiore has no "fear of AIDS"—she doesn't have HIV . . .
> She has since had two children . . . whom she boasted . . .
> have never been tested . . . But of course, Maggiore doesn't
> want them to be tested: she knows they are not at risk and

---

* One wonders how it is possible for anyone to refer to the questioning of the HIV/AIDS paradigm as "lucrative," as many people who have questioned this dogma have actually been harmed financially and career-wise.

their being uninfected would lead people to question her own status.[90]

Amazingly, last year a tragedy occurred that managed, in a moment, to change the public view of Christine's "status" from negative to positive.

In May 2005,[†] Eliza Jane, then three years old, came down with a cold that turned into an ear infection. After consultation with three doctors, she was prescribed Amoxicillin, which was taken in a dose exceeding that normally given to a child her size. She began throwing up, and within twenty-four hours she stopped breathing. After several hours of attempting to resuscitate her at the hospital, she died of cardiac arrest.

Within several months, the Los Angeles County coroner was informed that Christine was HIV-positive, and an investigation was undertaken into what previously had been a death for which AIDS was not even considered as a cause. Four months after Eliza Jane's death, the Los Angeles County coroner released a report stating that she died of AIDS-related pneumonia and HIV-induced encephalitis. This finding was supported by finding *Pneumocystis* in her lungs—although this is a ubiquitous organism present in over 90 percent of humans—and the HIV-associated core protein p24 in her brain (although not in her blood). Mysteriously, no HIV test results were released, although supposedly an HIV test was performed.

The parents hired another pathologist to perform a differential diagnosis, and he did so with the conclusion that she died of an allergic reaction to Amoxicillin. Nevertheless, the debate raged on,

---

†   Bergman's *New York Press* article was published in June 2005, implying that it must have been submitted before Bergman was aware of Eliza Jane's death, and certainly before its cause was ever questioned, in September 2005.

especially on various blog sites, with people attacking the credentials of the doctor who performed the differential diagnosis and attacking Christine (though not her husband, although presumably he had equal say in his child's healthcare decisions).

Recently, a story was published in the *Los Angeles CityBeat* in which the Eliza Jane Scovill case was extensively examined. One crucial piece of evidence was presented: Eliza Jane had an absolute lymphocyte count that was elevated, going completely against the government's definition of AIDS as a state of HIV-induced immune suppression.[91] That should have been the end of it, but it wasn't. The debate rages on.

This story is fascinating because it encapsulates everything that has come to characterize the AIDS debate, and all that is mysterious and ill-defined about the syndrome itself: a mother whose HIV status changes in people's minds according to whatever is convenient for them to think at the time; a death from PCP that exhibits absolutely no symptoms, even a day before her death; a diagnosis of AIDS made in spite of no HIV test results at all; and, saddest of all, vultures who will stop at nothing to prop up their paradigm, attacking a family who ought to have been left alone and ought always to have been left alone. There is no precedent for assuming that anyone but her parents has the right to decide on her health care, and as such there is no reason for any of us to believe we have a right to vote on it.

CHAPTER 8

Where Do We Go from Here?

AIDS does not inevitably lead to death, especially if we suppress the co-factors that support the disease. It is very important to tell this to people who are infected. I think we should put the same weight now on the co-factors as we have on HIV. Psychological factors are critical in supporting immune function. If you suppress this psychological support by telling someone he's condemned to die, your words alone will have condemned them.

Luc Montagnier, co-discoverer of HIV,
Wikipedia main site

Even the co-discoverer of HIV acknowledges the dangers of uncritically promoting the HIV=AIDS=DEATH hypothesis. In order to prevent more deaths caused by inappropriate medical treatment and the psychological terror that accompanies an HIV diagnosis, we must fairly and honestly assess all the evidence.

There are several practical considerations. HIV tests are unacceptably unspecific, given the ramifications of a reactive result. Using proper isolation (and not just culturing methods to detect viral markers), we must rigorously verify the accuracy of these tests. The isolation experiments as proposed by prominent scientists would cost about $100,000 but despite the fact that this would be a drop in the bucket by AIDS research standards, no funding is forthcoming.

There urgently needs to be a proper debate in the scientific literature between the foremost establishment scientists and the best-credentialed dissenting ones. But the scientific ruling majority (note the intentional use of an oxymoron) refuses to even consider the possibility that they might be wrong, despite every indication to the contrary, and the top HIV scientists in the country continually refuse to participate in a debate with any "dissident."

The suppression of debate goes back to Peter Duesberg's very first criticisms of the HIV debate and Robert Gallo's refusal to entertain any such debate by literally running away. It continues to this day with slanderous accusations by leading scientists and a refusal to "dignify" the dissenting arguments by responding to or even acknowledging them.

Harvey Bialy recently challenged Dr. John Moore of Cornell University to a debate on the AIDS Wiki regarding the etiology of AIDS. Dr. Bialy's challenge was: "I will present one fully referenced (with PDF files that the moderator can hyperlink) challenge to your favorite and livelihood-sustaining hypothesis, and you can demolish my feeble arguments in the same fashion. We will continue this for one additional round, and then move on to the next challenge. I have maybe seven such challenges. At the end, we will have produced the first fully documented, real scientific debate on the cause of AIDS. Interesting that after twenty-five years none has ever been held before, Bob Gallo's promise in the *PNAS* in 1989 notwithstanding."

Rather than accepting this debate, Moore replied by stating: "Participating in any public forum with the likes of Bialy would give him a credibility that he does not merit. The science community does not 'debate' with the AIDS denialists, it treats them with the utter contempt that they deserve and exposes them for the charlatans that they are. Kindly do not send me any further communications on this or any related matter."

Moore unwittingly exposes the true motivations of the AIDS "science community" in his reply to Bialy. It is clear that Moore and his ilk only desire to "expose charlatans" within self-defined constraints; namely, in situations in which they are protected from ever having to defend their own viewpoint and through channels that support their interests in their paradigm.

Furthermore, his choice of language is illuminating. He refers to the "scientific community," as though it were some sort of moral majority in-crowd, as though dissenters were not scientists at all— despite the fact that signatories to the petition for the Scientific Reappraisal of the HIV/AIDS Hypothesis number in the thousands and include two Nobel Prize winners and hundreds of PhDs and MDs. In Moore's view, apparently, none of these people qualifies as being a member of the "scientific community."

But HIV/AIDS research has always suffered from this sort of moral absolutism, outright discrimination, and suppression of argument. As Kary Mullis says in his book *Dancing Naked in the Mind Field*, "What people call science today is probably very similar to what we called science in 1634. Galileo was told to recant his beliefs or be excommunicated. People who refuse to accept the commandments of the AIDS establishment are basically told the same thing."[92]

The HIV theory has never been about science but rather about behavior modification primarily and, to a lesser extent, about money, power, and prestige. Language surrounding HIV and AIDS is infected with a sort of pious moralism that is completely inappropriate in science, and this sort of language is not restricted to the cultural and sociological aspects of AIDS. We can see it in the use of terms like "denialist" by scientists like Moore, and in the words of Dr. Mark Wainberg, who said that HIV dissenters are "perpetrators of death" and that "Peter Duesberg is the closest thing we have on this planet to a scientific sociopath."[93]

This same sort of science-by-majority-rule attitude can be seen in the words of an unnamed Berkeley scientist, interviewed by Celia Farber for her recent book, *Serious Adverse Events: An uncensored history of AIDS*: "He did it to himself, you know. You see, he wouldn't give up an idea. He went after it with a hammer. He may well be 3000 percent right, but he upset an awful lot of people . . . Nobody believed in him because what he was doing was overturning generally held views. They felt betrayed . . . You don't just stand up and say everybody is wrong."[63]

That sentence alone should illuminate just how much is wrong in HIV/AIDS science. But a society that has been so largely secularized has to believe in something with total faith, and for so many of us who don't have the time to look into the minutiae of every issue for ourselves, that something so often is science and scientific discoveries, broadcast to us in the reassuring tones of *those who know better*. We don't question—we have faith. As Mullis says about the high priests of science: "Thank your lucky stars that they didn't bother to change their clothes or their habits. They still wear priestly white robes and they don't do heavy labor. It makes them easier to spot."

In his 1993 book *Rethinking AIDS: The Tragic Cost of Premature Consensus*, Robert Root-Bernstein wrote: "We do not understand AIDS." Fifteen years later, we still do not understand AIDS. And we will *never* understand AIDS until we acknowledge our own ignorance, but there are powerful forces at work preventing such acknowledgment.

First of all, there are tremendous financial and social interests involved. Billions of dollars in research funding, stock options, and activist budgets are predicated on the assumption that HIV causes AIDS. Entire industries of pharmaceutical drugs, diagnostic testing, and activist causes would have no reason to exist.

Second, the scientific and medical communities have a great deal of face to lose. It is not much of an exaggeration to state that when the HIV/AIDS hypothesis is finally recognized as wrong, the entire institution of science will lose the public's trust, and science itself will experience fundamental, profound, and long-lasting changes. The "scientific community" has risked its credibility by standing by the HIV theory for so long. This is why doubting the HIV hypothesis is now tantamount to doubting science itself, and this is why dissidents face excommunication.

Third, doctors have become emotionally attached to the idea of an HIV/AIDS pandemic threatening to take over the world. The HIV/AIDS "predictions" are a projection of the medical profession's self-identity, and taking away the HIV/AIDS paradigm threatens the medical profession's self-identity.[94]

Fourth, powerful psychological forces are at work. It is simply easier for most people to project our neglect of disenfranchised groups—gay men, drug users, blacks, the poor, and so on—onto a virus and accept those "infected" as sacrificial victims, than to recognize that *there is no bug*. For society, the latter would require acceptance of these disenfranchised groups as equal participants in mainstream society and culture.

However, the most significant obstacle of all is apathy. In a world full of constant distraction, most people are content to live in the public reality created by the media and advertisers. They do not want to be disturbed or provoked. Our most important goal is to make people *care*. We must reach their hearts, as well as their minds, and appeal to their inherent sense of justice and of what is right and wrong.

At this point, it is up to each person to acknowledge their own ignorance, to do their own homework, and to decide for themselves. To make that decision, all information must be available to everyone because, after all, as we have been told from the beginning by the AIDS mainstream, SILENCE=DEATH.

Afterword

A Roadmap for Future Action

If we could succeed and lock a couple of these guys up, I guarantee you the HIV-denier movement would die pretty darn quickly.

—Dr. Mark Wainberg, 2000

It is sometimes nearly impossible to separate science from propaganda in AIDS. Totalitarian scientific propaganda requires repetition and the illusion of consistency.

—Charles Ortleb, personal communication with author

The late Dr. Mark Wainberg openly called for the criminal conviction of anyone who publicly questions the HIV/AIDS hypothesis. In case anyone wondered what the state of intellectual and scientific debate is in this so called progressive, enlightened time, I refer you to the quote above. Twenty-two years later, having witnessed the deplatforming of scientists and journalists who dared question even the COVID *response,* we can see that things have not improved. They may be even worse.

We do not live in a time that scientific debate is encouraged. Rather, science in general, and medical science in particular, are beholden to governmental regulatory agencies and to pharmaceutical interests. Any question of the prevailing consensus is swiftly dealt with by ruthless campaigns to paint the questioner as either a lunatic or a danger to society.

When the original version of this volume was published, I was employed as an assistant professor at The University of Texas at Tyler, and had a promising publication list in addition to being actively involved in peer review of mathematical and biomathematical research, having been on the editorial board of the *Journal of Biological Systems.*

Upon publication, some very strange things occurred. Letters began pouring in to the president of my university, warning him that I was a dangerous menace to society that threatened the integrity of the institution at which I was employed. About two dozen such letters were sent. They all said much the same thing, which led me to believe that this was a coordinated attack.

One curiosity of these so called "warnings" was that several of them stated—falsely—that I had been giving medical advice to AIDS patients online. This was absolutely false, and something I would never do, but the truth was even stranger. It turned out that someone or someones (I never figured out who) was in fact *posing as me* online, and giving medical advice to people who identified as AIDS patients, presumably anticipating that it was actually me acting in a highly unethical manner. Furthermore, there were a number of situations in which an AIDS activist actually tracked down and phoned my husband hoping to get "the dirt" on me, but the so-called AIDS activist never identified him or herself.

Eventually the pressure must have proven too much, as without warning, I was told that my contract would not be renewed. No reason was given—untenured faculty can be terminated at any time for any reason and *no reason need be given.* I was given the reason that my publication rate had "dropped off," despite that at the time I had more publications than any faculty member below the rank of full professor. To be clear, I *don't know* what circumstances or conversations actually occurred behind the scenes.

I can't say for sure that I was fired because of my heterodox views on HIV. I can only speculate, and my speculations may be incorrect. I don't pretend to be a mind reader. What I can see is that the past few years have shone a very bright light on the fact that *many* researchers, doctors, and scientists can *very easily* be "cancelled" for not walking in lockstep with the prevailing, government-endorsed consensus.

Returning to the case of HIV, I will point out something that needs to be very strongly emphasized, and that is that when AIDS came onto the scene, retrovirology was a field in its infancy. In the 1980s, scientists were not aware of the ubiquity of retroviruses and retroviral genetic sequences, let alone the potential for endogenous retroviruses to be involved in disease states. It was an exciting new field, and one of the dangers of working in an exciting new field is the temptation to see everything from the perspective of that field. Thus it was that the search for a pathogen that was tropic for CD4+ T cells led to an extremely narrow focus on a retrovirus that could potentially cause damage to these cells, effectively ignoring any other cellular disruptions and any other viruses in AIDS; ironic considering AIDS was characterized by *many* opportunistic infections, some of which were caused by viruses. I cannot over-state how the prevailing research climate at the time was primed to make a "rookie mistake," the mistake in this case being the laser focus on CD4+ T cells and the alleged retrovirus HIV. Had this syndrome emerged at a later time, perhaps things would have been very different. Consider also the prevailing attitude toward homo-sexuality in the 1980s. Homosexuals and especially gay men were heavily discriminated against, to the point that the concept of "risk groups" emerged very quickly, having the net effect of making any-one *not* in a risk group believe that they didn't need to worry about the issue. It fades from concern as people in these so called risk groups are ghettoized and used as guinea pigs for drug regimes that are quite extreme and of dubious safety.

Indeed, the "HIV causes AIDS by drastically reducing levels of CD4+ T cells" model of causation appears to be quietly falling out of favor. The focus seems to have moved to the idea that HIV causes disease by inducing massive inflammation, which leads to cardiovascular disease and neoplasms. This is curious because AIDS is meant to be a disease of *immune deficiency*, but switch-ing the focus to inflammation implies that there is actually some immune *over*-activation occurring, as well.

Furthermore, had researchers been looking for an agent capable of causing massive inflammation back in the early 1980s, would HIV have even been considered a viable suspect?

Endless repetition of phrases such as "know your status," "undetectable = untransmissible," "HIV disease," "the virus that causes AIDS," and "lifesaving drugs" happens so often they become accepted simply because we are so used to hearing them. It doesn't matter if they are true. One of the best ways to sell a lie is to repeat it over and over again until it has been subliminally accepted by most people. Doctors are no exception. The average general practitioner does not have time to read all the medical literature, especially if they are not a specialist in a particular subfield of medicine. They necessarily must rely on the CDC, the NIH, and similar government agencies for information to inform their practices, but if these agencies are corrupt or beholden to larger financial interests, the quality of the information they provide is irreparably compromised.

It is long past time for a regime change. If this volume has done nothing else, I hope that it inspires people to know that we have been given a window of opportunity for a new level of honesty and transparency in scientific research in general, and AIDS in particular. The purpose of this short afterword is to provide concrete steps that can be taken to get, once and for all, real answers to the epidemic of immune dysregulation that includes, but is not limited to AIDS.

I include two lists here. The first is political and scientific and the second is psychosocial.

- There need to be congressional hearings that honestly and thoroughly examine the history of fraud and incompetence in AIDS research.
- We must launch a Reproducibility Project in AIDS research. At a minimum, the Gallo et al papers from 1984 and the Ho/Wei and Ho/Shaw papers from 1995–96 need to be critically examined and retracted by both *Science* and *Nature* if found not to be reproducible. It is possible that *every* scientific paper promoting the role of HIV in AIDS should be retracted.
- Class action lawyers need to be retained to obtain restitution for individuals who have been harmed by defective

products such as the HIV antibody tests and the viral load test.

- Class action lawyers also must be retained to obtain compensation for people who have been harmed by so-called anti-HIV drugs. This is already happening.

- AIDS research funding needs to be freed from the chokehold of the laser focus on HIV. Specifically, funding must immediately be made available to study the issues of non-HIV AIDS; endogenous retroviruses that encode superantigens, other viruses like HHV-6 and EBV that are known to be harmful in AIDS, including non-HIV AIDS, and alternative treatment modalities.

- All awards given for HIV research should be retracted, including a posthumous retraction of Montagnier's Nobel.

Unfortunately, none of these things will be possible without the cooperation and enlightenment of certain groups of people—those who promote the HIV hypothesis of AIDS and those who are victimized by it.

- The journalism and media communities in general need to widen their focus and reconsider their lockstep repetition of the pronouncements of public health authorities. Journalists need to be allowed to ask difficult questions without fear of censorship or worse. Journalists must not be afraid to question any official narrative, but must instead return to traditional investigative journalism rather than the empty sock puppet role of simply repeating the "official story" handed them by government officials like some kind of echo chamber.

- Journalists (and in my fantasy world, everyone) need to quit being dazzled and confused by mathematical and computer models and develop critical thinking skills and a minimal level of numeracy that would enable them to critically examine any mathematical and statistical claims, rather than accepting them with blind faith.

- The gay community, or at least large swaths of this community, needs to recognize that they are victims of a kind of Stockholm Syndrome at the hands of AIDS activists and the pharmaceutical industry. This kind of shift is challenging because it is difficult for *anyone* to admit that they've unwittingly participated in their own victimization. But it must happen, or many more will be imprisoned by a bankrupt paradigm and, worse, if the PrEP pushers get their way, become guinea pigs in the potentially disastrous public health experiment that basically amounts to using "HIV drugs" as HIV *vaccines,* making them customers of Big Pharma for life, even if they have no hint of HIV.

- The African American community must be reminded of the Tuskegee syphilis experiment and the AIDS drug trials at the Incarnation Children's Center. They need to understand that the focus on communities of color is not benevolent but sinister, and attempts to make them the target of human rights violations reminiscent of Tuskegee. The African American community, as well as the gay community, needs to know that the public health bureaucrats and the pharmaceutical industry are *not* their friends.

The HIV hypothesis of AIDS is undoubtedly harmful to those who are unfortunate enough to get caught up in the web of testing and unending toxic treatments, not to mention the stigma and "othering" associated with a designation of HIV-positive.

That is merely the tip of the iceberg when it comes to the harm that has been done in the name of defending a hypothesis that has produced many excuses but no explanations. The designation of the "risk groups" neatly ghettoized said risk groups from the very beginning, while creating a false sense of security in those not in the risk groups.

The attempt to follow the scientific method has been sabotaged at every turn. Knee jerk suppression of dissent from the start—far before there was any level of certainty regarding AIDS causation—has prevented any real progress. The hostile and demeaning attitude of those like the late Dr. Wainberg and his wish to criminalize HIV dissent is entirely unprofessional, and it is everywhere present. I am not being dramatic when I say that the field of AIDS research is effectively a toxic work environment at this point. If it weren't so tragic it would be funny.

The scientific and medical communities have a great deal of face to lose. The "scientific community" has risked its credibility by standing by the HIV theory for so long, and this mistake is now coming home to roost, as the mismanagement of COVID the world over has opened many eyes to the fact that the scientific community is not always objective and quite often has its own agenda that has nothing to do with the search for truth.

Failed Predictions of the HIV/AIDS Hypothesis

In order to be considered viable, any scientific hypothesis needs to do two things—explain and predict. If a hypothesis finds itself, time and time again, making predictions that fail, it either needs to be seriously reassessed or to be considered a failed hypothesis.

Consider just a few of the predictions made by the HIV hypothesis of AIDS and decide for yourself.

- **HIV causes immune deficiency by killing CD4+ T-cells.** In fact, it is currently not believed that HIV kills T-cells in any way, but rather, that HIV primes T-cells to commit suicide at some later time. This hypothesis has been put forward to explain the lack of evidence for any cell-killing mechanism that can be attributed to HIV. Furthermore, in a peculiar pivot, the focus seems to be changing from the

"HIV-mediated loss of CD4+ T cells" to the idea of "HIV-mediated inflammation," which is strange indeed considering inflammation is typically considered to be immune *over*activation, rather than extreme immune suppression that has always been considered the hallmark of "HIV disease."

- **HIV will spread rapidly through the population.** "If the spread of AIDS continues at this rate, in 1996 there could be one billion people infected; five years later, hypothetically ten billion... Could we be facing the threat of extinction during our lifetime?" —Theresa Crenshaw, President's AIDS Commission, 1987. Currently only *38 million* people worldwide are estimated to be HIV-positive, which is significantly fewer than was predicted at the beginning of the "epidemic." Furthermore, as the HIV prevalence curve and the CDC's own data show, at least in the US, HIV has not spread at all since testing was first available.

- **By 1990, one in five heterosexuals may be dead of AIDS.** This prediction, made in 1987, has proved catastrophically wrong. Approximately one in 250 Americans is estimated to test HIV-positive, and outside the risk groups this number drops to about one in *five thousand*—a far cry from the "one in five" figure cited in 1987.

- **AIDS will decimate Africa.** But even in the hardest-hit regions of sub-Saharan Africa, the population is growing at a rate of a few percent per year. HIV estimates are derived from extrapolation of data obtained by anonymously testing the blood of pregnant women with a single ELISA test. Since the beginning of the AIDS era, the population of Africa has increased by nearly 300 million—an increase equal to the entire population of the United States.

- **A cure will be available by 1986.** This pronouncement was made at the Gallo-Heckler April 1984 press conference. Not only has it failed absolutely, it is now acknowledged that a cure is unlikely to ever be found. As Dr. Joe Sonnabend has said, "The notion of 'eradication' is just total science fiction. The RNA of retroviruses turns into DNA and becomes part of us. It's part of our being. You can't ever get rid of it" (Farber 2000).

- **A vaccine will be available by 1986.** This pronouncement was made at the same press conference that so boldly predicted a cure. Not only has every vaccine trial to date been a flop, a vaccine may be impossible since HIV-positive individuals all have antibody to HIV already. There are therefore two options—either having antibodies is not protective, in which case a Jennerian vaccine is useless; or having antibodies is protective, in which case HIV is harmless and no vaccine is needed.

- **HIV will spread primarily by sexual transmission, needlestick injuries, and needle-sharing drug use.** Since only one in a thousand unprotected sexual contacts with an HIV-positive person is estimated to transmit HIV, even a constant number of cases could not be sustained in this way. Clearly, the dominant mode of HIV transmission must be other than sexual. However, to date fewer than one hundred needle-stick transmissions of HIV have even been reported. Additionally, studies show that users of needle-exchange programs are significantly *more* likely to test HIV-positive than those who do not use clean needles.

- **If HIV is the sole cause of AIDS, it must be present at high titer in AIDS patients and conversely, AIDS will not be present in the HIV-negative.** HIV has proven barely to be found in AIDS patients. in fact, according to Gallo's original research, HIV was found with higher frequency in pre-AIDS patients (at 88 percent) than in AIDS patients (at 36 percent). Viral load is only measured using PCR since many HIV-positive individuals have no evidence of virus by culture. By contrast, traditional viruses such as herpes, influenza, smallpox, etc. only cause disease at very high titer—thousands or millions of infectious units per cubic millimeter of infected tissue. As far as finding no AIDS in the HIV-free, this idea was rendered obsolete with the addition of ICL in 1993 to explain the "HIV-free AIDS" cases that appeared and continue to appear.

- **AIDS will develop within one to five years from infection with HIV.** This prediction, made in the mid-1980s, has had to be changed several times to avoid the embarrassment of explaining exactly why it is that AIDS rarely develops within such a short time frame. By 1998 the latent period had been estimated to be ten to fifteen years, and at the current time it is claimed to be about ten years, but little is known as to how accurate that is. Furthermore, it presents a conundrum when one considers the first AIDS cases: If AIDS takes ten years, on average, to appear, then we should expect that these original AIDS patients were all *at least* thirty or so years old. But many of the first AIDS patients were in their early twenties (ages ranged from early twenties to the late forties among the first hundred men with AIDS), leaving as HIV believer with no other option than to consider that they became infected at twelve or thirteen years of age.

- **AIDS does not discriminate.** However, in Europe and the US, AIDS remains restricted to the risk groups of homosexuals and drug abusers. The vast majority of cases affect men, and those not in the risk groups rarely develop AIDS without profoundly immunosuppressive cofactors such as hemophilia or antiviral therapy. Even more damning is the fact that different risk groups exhibit different AIDS-defining diseases (Duesberg 1992).

- **Anti-HIV drugs stop AIDS.** The annual mortality rate of HIV-positives undergoing antiviral therapy is much higher, at 7 to 9 percent, than the mortality rate of all HIV-positives worldwide, at about 1 to 2 percent per year (Duesberg, Koehnlein, and Rasnick 2003a). Furthermore, there is ample evidence that treated HIV-positives die much faster of liver failure or cardiac failure than they would have had they developed AIDS in the first place. Also, it is estimated that approximately one-third of HIV-positives, even in the US, do not know their status. If this is the case, there should be a huge number of people dying suddenly of AIDS, and this is not happening.

- **AIDS, and HIV, will spread randomly.** This is clearly not the case. AIDS remains restricted largely to the risk groups, and HIV itself is dramatically more common among people of African descent than among Asians or Caucasians. HIV theorists have invented convoluted explanations for why this is so. The most popular is currently that a nontrivial proportion of Caucasians possess a CCR-delta receptor deletion, rendering them immune to HIV. Supposedly neither Asians nor Africans possess this mutation. This theory does nothing to explain why it is that the incidence of HIV is in fact lower among Asians than it is among Caucasians, nor does it explain why large populations of African prostitutes in high-risk areas such as Nairobi appear to be immune to HIV.

- **The prostitution and pornography industries will be decimated by AIDS.** But prostitutes are not at risk for AIDS unless they are also drug users, and there are virtually no clients who have contracted AIDS from a prostitute. Moreover, the porn industry remains largely unaffected despite the fact that condoms are rarely used and testing is known to be inaccurate.

Suggested Further Reading/Viewing

- *The Logic of Scientific Discovery*, Karl Popper
- *The Structure of Scientific Revolutions*, Thomas Kuhn
- *The Knowledge Machine: How Irrationality Created Modern Science*, Michael Strevens
- *Osler's Web: Inside the Labyrinth of the Chronic Fatigue Syndrome Epidemic*, Hillary Johnson
- *The Chronic Fatigue Syndrome Epidemic Cover-up: How a little newspaper solved the biggest scientific and political mystery of our time*, Charles Ortleb
- *Poison by Prescription: The AZT Story*, John Lauritsen
- *The AIDS War*, John Lauritsen
- *Infectious AIDS: Have we Been Misled?* Peter Duesberg
- *Inventing the AIDS Virus*, Peter Duesberg
- *AIDS: The Failure of Contemporary Science*, Neville Hodgkinson
- *What if Everything You Thought You Knew about AIDS Was Wrong?* Christine Maggiore

- *Oncogenes, Aneuploidy, and AIDS*, Harvey Bialy
- *Serious Adverse Events: An Uncensored History of AIDS*, Celia Farber
- *When AIDS Began*, Michelle Cochrane
- *Rethinking AIDS: The Tragic Cost of Premature Consensus*, Robert Root-Bernstein
- *Debating AZT*, Anthony Brink
- *Dancing Naked in the Mind Field*, Kary Mullis
- *Wrongful Death: The AIDS Trial*, Stephen Davis
- *The Other Side of AIDS*, directed by Robin Scovill
- *The Last Lovers on Earth*, directed by Charles Ortleb

Glossary

ad hominem: A form of arguing in which the strategy is to attack the person presenting the argument rather than the substance of the argument itself.

AIDS: Acquired Immune Deficiency Syndrome, a classification consisting of any one of twenty-five to thirty different medical conditions plus positive antibody to HIV. The term AIDS replaced GRID in 1982.

AIDS-phobia: A term coined to describe the phenomenon wherein people who had recently had close contact with someone they suspected to be HIV-positive exhibited some symptoms of AIDS despite persistently testing HIV-negative.

Amoxicillin: A moderate-spectrum antibiotic used to inhibit a variety of gram-positive, and some gram-negative, bacteria.

antibody: A protein that is meant to identify and neutralize foreign objects such as viruses and bacteria.

antibody test: A laboratory test, usually performed on blood and sometimes on other bodily fluids such as saliva, that tests for the presence of antibodies to a particular organism by determining whether there is a reaction between the bodily fluid and certain antigens in the test kit. These antigens should be specific to the pathogen for which it is being tested.

antigen: A substance that initiates antibody production.

apoptosis: A type of programmed cell death, in which cells destroy themselves deliberately.

CD4+ T-cells: A subset of the lymphocytes involved in activating and directing other immune cells. Also called helper T-cells, CD4+ T-cells do not kill or destroy pathogens themselves.

cell-mediated immunity: The branch of the immune system that handles intracellular parasites, such as viruses, fungi, and myco-bacteria. Some consider cell-mediated immunity to have some involvement in cancer surveillance.

correlation: A measure of the strength of the association between two or more variables. Correlation does not necessarily indicate a causal relationship between the variables.

differential diagnosis: Essentially a "second opinion"; when a person's initial diagnosis is inconsistent with clinical symptoms and a new diagnosis is sought, the new diagnosis is the differential diagnosis.

electron micrograph: A photograph or image taken through an electron microscope (a very high-powered microscope used to detect items too small to be seen via ordinary microscope) to show a magnified image of an item.

ELISA: The enzyme-linked immunosorbent assay is a technique used to detect the presence of antibody or antigen in a sample. It uses two antibodies, the first of which is specific to the antigen and the second of which is coupled to an enzyme (this second antibody gives the assay its "enzyme-linked" name) and will cause a chromatogenic or fluorogenic substrate to produce a signal, which is seen as a color change.

endogenous: A factor or factors that originate from within an organism, e.g. the hormone estrogen is synthesized endogenously.

epidemiology: The branch of science concerned with factors affecting the health of individuals and populations.

etiology: Related to the causation of disease.

exogenous: A factor or factors that originate from outside an organism; e.g., medication taken intravenously is exogenous.

genome: The hereditary information of an organism, encoded in their DNA or RNA.

GRID: The original name for AIDS, dating from 1980; the acronym stands for Gay-Related Immune Deficiency.

HAART: Highly Active AntiRetroviral Therapy refers to a combination of three or four antiretroviral drugs given to HIV-positives.

HIV: An acronym that stands for Human Immunodeficiency Virus. HIV replaced the American term "HTLV-III" and the French term "LAV" to describe phenomena attributed to an exogenous retrovirus, often found in AIDS patients and commonly considered the causative agent of AIDS.

humoral immunity: The branch of the immune system that handles extracellular parasites such as bacteria and worms. It is also involved in antibody production.

hypergammaglobulinemia: A condition in which an individual's immune system produces too many antibodies to both internal and external antigens.

hypothesis: A suggested explanation of some phenomena.

immune system: A system of specialized cells and organs that protect the organism from biological influences (mostly exogenous).

immunology: The branch of biological science that studies all aspects of the immune system in all organisms.

isolation: The separation of a biological agent from any other agent; removal of contaminants.

Koch's postulates: Four criteria published by Robert Koch in 1890, used to establish a causal relationship between organism and disease. These are (1) the organism must be found in all individuals suffering from the disease, and in no healthy individuals; (2) the organism must be isolated from a diseased individual and grown in pure culture; (3) the cultured organism should cause disease when introduced into a healthy individual; and (4) the organism must then be reisolated from the experimentally infected individual.

lymphadenopathy: Abnormal swelling of the lymph nodes.

lymphocyte: Any of a number of white blood cells in the immune system involved in the defense against pathogens.

lymphocytopenia: Also called lymphopenia, a condition characterized by a marked depression in the number of lymphocytes.

mathematical biology: A field of study that models natural and biological processes using deterministic and stochastic predictive systems. The field includes models of population dynamics, cell biology, ecology, and physiological systems. This is not to be confused with statistical modeling, which analyzes biological systems using data.

mitogen: A chemical that prompts a cell to begin cell division (mitosis).

opportunistic infection: An infection caused by an organism that does not usually harm an individual with a healthy immune system but may cause disease in an immune-suppressed host.

paradigm: A thought pattern in a scientific or epistemological context.

pathogen: A biological agent that causes disease or illness in its host.

polymerase chain reaction (PCR): A method of amplifying (mass producing) DNA so it can be seen more easily.

positive predictive value (PPV): The PPV of a test indicates the proportion of positive tests that can be expected to indicate the true prevalence of the pathogen being tested for in a target population. For example, a 100 percent PPV means that every positive test is a true positive, whereas a 10 percent PPV means that only 10 percent of the positive tests are true positives, and that 90 percent of positive tests are false positives.

prevalence: Defined to be the ratio of the number of people in a population affected by a certain disease to the total number of susceptible people in the population.

protease inhibitor: A type of medication that inhibits viral protease, an enzyme used by viruses to assemble new viruses.

retrovirus: An enveloped virus possessing an RNA genome, which replicates via reverse transcription. RNA is transcribed into DNA using the enzyme reverse transcriptase and is then incorporated into the host cell's genome via the integrase enzyme.

reverse transcriptase: Also known as RNA-directed DNA polymerase. A DNA polymerase enzyme that transcribes single-strand RNA into double-strand DNA, the reverse of the way transcription normally occurs.

sensitivity: A measure of how likely it is that a particular test will produce a negative result when in fact the true result is positive. The better the sensitivity, the fewer false negatives will occur.

specificity: A measure of how likely it is that a test will produce a positive result when in fact the true result is negative. A highly specific test will yield few false positives.

teratogen: An adverse circumstance, including a variety of substances that cause congenital malformations in fetuses and babies.

viral load: A term meant to indicate the number of infectious viruses in a given sample of tissue. The HIV viral load uses quantitative PCR to magnify and estimate the number of HIV-associated RNA fragments in a milliliter of blood. Official estimates (Piatak Jr. et al. 1993) consider HIV viral loads to overestimate infectious virus titers by a factor of 60,000. Viral load is not used to diagnose HIV infection.

Western Blot test (WB): Also called an immunoblot, the WB is a method used to detect protein in a sample. The WB uses gel electrophoresis to separate proteins according to molecular weight and then determines the strength of sample reactions against these proteins individually rather than as a mixture.

Endnotes

1. Wikipedia contributors, "Tuskegee Syphilis Study." 2022. [Online]. Available: https://en.wikipedia.org/wiki/Tuskegee_Syphilis_Study
2. T. Miller, "CDC, NIH, Condemn 'Deeply Saddening' Guatemala Study." 2010. [Online]. Available: https://pbs.org/newshour/health/cdc-nih-condemn -deeply-saddening-guatemala-study
3. L. Scheff, "The house that AIDS built." 2004. [Online]. Available: http://www.altheal.org/toxicity/house.html
4. J. Kastner, "Drugmaker accused of withholding safer meds from HIV patients, San Diego man speaks out." 2021.
5. C. Mendoza, A. Holguin, and V. Soriano, "False positives for HIV using commercial viral load quantification," *AIDS*, vol. 11812(15), pp. 2076–2077, 1998.
6. H. Bauer, "Demographic characteristics of HIV II: What determines the frequence of positive HIV tests?" *Journal of Scientific Exploration*, vol. 20, pp. 69–94, 2006.
7. R. C. Gallo et al., "Frequent detection and isolation of cytopathis retroviruses (HTLV-III) from patients with AIDS and at risk for AIDS," *Science*, vol. 224, pp. 500–502, 1984.
8. R. Giraldo, "Everyone reacts positive on the ELISA test for HIV," *Continuum*, vol. 5(5), pp. 8–11, 1998.
9. D. D. Ho, A. U. Neumann, A. S. Perelson, W. Chen, J. M. Leonard, and M. Markowitz, "Rapid turnover of plasma virions and CD4 lymphocytes in HIV-1 infection," *Nature*, vol. 373, pp. 123–126, 1995.

10. X. Wei et al., "Viral dynamics in human immunodeficiency virus type 1 infection," *Nature*, vol. 373, pp. 117–122, 1995.

11. A. United, "Ending the HIV Epidemic in the United States: A roadmap for federal action." 2022. [Online]. Available: https://viventhealth.org/wp-content/uploads/2021/02/Ending_the_HIV_Epidemic_in_the_United_States__-11.pdf

12. Gilead, "State of the HIV Epidemic." [Online]. Available: https://gileadhiv.com/landscape/state-of-epidemic

13. R. Grant, J. Lama, P. Anderson, and et al., "Preexposure Chemoprophylaxis for HIV Prevention in Men who Have Sex with Men," *N. Engl. J. Med.*, vol. 363, pp. 2587–2599, 2010.

14. M. Deutsch, D. Glidden, J. Sevelius, and et al., "HIV pre-exposure prophylaxis in transgender women: a subgroup analysis of the iPrEx trial," *Lancet HIV*, vol. 2(12), pp. 512–9, 2015.

15. J. Baeten, D. Donnell, P. Ndase, and et al., "Antiretroviral Prophylaxis for HIV Prevention in Heterosexual Men and Women," *N. Engl. J. Med.*, no. 367, pp. 399-410., 2012.

16. K. Choopanya, M. Martin, P. Suntharasamai, and et al., "Antiretroviral prophylaxis for HIV infection in injecting drug users in Bangkok, Thailand (The Bangkok Tenofovir Study): a randomised, double-blind, placebo-controlled phase 3 trial," *The Lancet*, no. 381(9883), pp. 2083–2090, 2013.

17. H. Bauer, "Demographic characteristics of HIV I: How did HIV spread?" *Journal of Scientific Exploration*, vol. 19, pp. 567–603, 2005.

18. R. Eisinger, C. Dieffenbach, and A. Fauci, "HIV Viral Load and Transmissibility of HIV Infection: Undetectable Equals Untransmittable," *JAMA*, vol. 321(5), pp. 451–452, 2019.

19. N.-'t Hoen, E., T. Cremer, R. Gallo, and L. Margolis, "Extracellular vesicles and viruses: Are they close relatives?" *PNAS*, vol. 113(33), pp. 9155–9161, 2016.

20. B. De La Hera et al., "Role of the human endogenous retrovirus HERV-K18 in autoimmune disease susceptibility: study in the Spanish population and meta-analysis," *PLoS One*, vol. 8, 2013.

21. P. Duesberg, C. Koehnlein, and D. Rasnick, "Incidence of AIDS in the U.S. Population." 2003. [Online]. Available: http://rethinkaids.info/graphs.htm

22. CDC, "HIV/AIDS Surveillance Report," no. 15. pp. 1–46, 2004.

23. CDC, "HIV prevalence, unrecognized infection, and HIV testing among men who have sex with men: Five U.S. cities, June 2004-April 2005," *MMWR*, no. 54. 2005.

24. P. Duesberg, C. Koehnlein, and D. Rasnick, "The chemical bases of the various AIDS epidemics: Recreational drugs, antiviral chemotherapy, and malnutrition," *J. Biosci.*, vol. 28, pp. 383–412, 2003.

25. J. Crewdson, *Science Fictions: A Scientific Mystery, a Massive Cover-up and the Dark Legacy of Robert Gallo*. Little, Brown., 2003.

26. R. Strohman, "Preface to *Infectious AIDS: Have we been misled?*"

27. NIH, "The evidence that HIV causes AIDS." 2003. [Online]. Available: http://www.niaid.nih.gov/factsheets/evidhiv.htm"

28. "The Durban Declaration," *Nature*, vol. 406, no. 6791, pp. 15–16, 2000.

29. R. Johnston, M. Irwin, and D. Crowe, "Durban Declaration Rebuttal." 2001. [Online]. Available: http://www.rethinkaids.info/durbandeclaration rebuttal.htm"

30. E. de Harven, "Retroviruses: The recollections of an electron microscopist," *Reappraising AIDS*, no. 6(11), pp. 4–7, 1998.

31. M. Craddock, "HIV: Science by press conference," in *AIDS: Virus or Drug Induced?* pp. 127–30.

32. H. Bialy, "Oncogenes, Aneuploidy, and AIDS," Berkeley, CA: North Atlantic Books, 2004.

33. J. Embretson et al., "Massive covert infection of helper T lymphocytes and macrophages by HIV during the incubation period of AIDS," *Nature*, vol. 362, pp. 359–62, 1993.

34. G. Pantaleo et al., "HIV infection is active and progressive in lymphoid tissue during the clinically latent state of disease," *Nature*, vol. 362, pp. 355–358, 1993.

35. E. Papadopulos-Eleopulos, V. F. Turner, J. M. Papadimitriou, D. Causer, B. Hedland-Thomas, and B. A. Page, "A critical analysis of the HIV-T4 cell-AIDS hypothesis," *Genetica*, vol. 95, pp. 5–24, 1995.

36. M. Piatak Jr. et al., "High levels of HIV-1 in plasma during all stages of infection determined by quantitative competitive PCR," *Science*, vol. 259, pp. 1749–1754, 1993.

37. P. Duesberg and H. Bialy, "Duesberg and the right of reply according to Maddox—Nature," in *AIDS: Virus or Drug Induced?* P. H. Duesberg, Ed. Dordrecht, Netherlands: Kluwer Academic Publishing, 1996, pp. 241–70.

38. M. Roederer, "Getting to the HAART of T cell dynamics," *Nature Medicine*, vol. 4, pp. 145–146, 1998.

39. J. Embretson et al., "Analysis of human immunodeficiency virus-infected tissues by amplification and in situ hybridization reveals latent and permissive infection at single-cell resolution," *Proc. Natl. Acad. Sci.*, vol. 90(1), pp. 357–61, 2003.

40. CDC, "Classification system for human T-lymphotropic virus type III/ lymphadenopthy-associated virus infections," *MMWR*, no. 35. p. 334, 1986.

41. D. Brown, "Twenty years ago today, doctors first warned the world of the emergence of a deadly new disease - AIDS," *Washington Post*, Jun. 2001.

42. CDC, "1993 Revised classification system for HIV infection and expanded surveillance case definition for AIDS among adolescents and adults," *MMWR*, no. 41. 1993.

43. M. Cochrane, *When AIDS Began: San Francisco and the Making of an Epidemic*. New York: Routledge, 2004.

44. E. Papadopulos-Eleopulos, V. F. Turner, J. M. Papadimitriou, and D. Causer, "Factor VIII, HIV and AIDS in haemophiliacs: An analysis of their relationship," *Genetica*, vol. 95, pp. 25–50, 1995.

45. P. Duesberg, "AIDS acquired by drug consumption and other noncontagious risk factors," *Pharmac. Ther.*, vol. 55, pp. 201–77, 1992.

46. J. S. Beck, R. C. Potts, T. Kardjito, and J. M. Grange, "T4 lymphopenia in patients with active pulmonary tuberculosis.," *Clin Exp Immunol*, vol. 60, pp. 49–54, 1985.

47. W. P. Carney, R. H. Rubin, R. A. Hoffman, W. P. Hansen, K. Healey, and M. S. Hirsch, "Analysis of T lymphocyte subsets in CMV mononucleaosis," *The Journal of Immunology*, no. 126(6), pp. 2114–16, 1981.

48. D. C. Des Jarlais et al., "Development of AIDS, HIV seroconversion, and potential cofactors for CD4 cell loss in a cohort of intravenous drug users," *AIDS*, vol. 1(2), pp. 105–11, 1987.

49. T. J. Verde, S. G. Thomas, R. W. Moore, P. Shek, and R. J. Shephard, "Immune responses and increased training of the elite athlete," *J Appl Physiol*, vol. 73, no. 4, pp. 1494–9, 1992.

50. J. Lauritsen, *Poison by Prescription, The AZT Story*. Pagan Press, 1990.

51. C. Atzori, E. Angeli, A. Mainini, F. Agostoni, V. Micheli, and A. Cargnel, "In vitro activity of human immunodeficiency virus protease inhibitors against Pneumocystis carinii," *Journal of Infectious Diseases*, vol. 181, no. 5, pp. 1629–34, 2000.

52. K. Anastos, Y. Barrón, and P. Miotti, "Risk of progression to AIDS and death in women infected with HIV-1 initiating highly active antitreviral treatment at different stages of disease," *Arch. Intern. Med.*, vol. 162, pp. 1973–80, 2002.

53. U. H. System, "Better monitoring of liver enzymes is needed to save lives of people with HIV," *Heal Toronto*, 2002. [Online]. Available: http://www .healthtoronto.com/justice_liver.html

54. S. R. Hosein, "Side effects: Causes of serious illness among HAART-users not clear." 2002. [Online]. Available: http://www.healtoronto.com /catie_14_3.html

55. A. Cassone, F. De Bernardis, A. Torosantucci, E. Tacconelli, M. Tumbarello, and R. Cauda, "In vitro and in vivo anticandidial activity of human immunodeficiency virus protease inhibitors," *Journal of Infectious Diseases*, no. 180(2), pp. 448–45, 1999.

56. R. Culshaw, "Why I Quit HIV: The Aftermath." 2006. [Online]. Available: http://www.LewRockwell.com/orig7/culshaw2.html

57. M. D. of P. Health, "Who is dying from HIV/AIDS and how has this changed over time." 2002. [Online]. Available: http://www.mass.gov/dph /aids/research/profile2002/word_doc/chap_7.doc

58. R. M. Cordes, "Pitfalls in HIV testing," *Postgraduate Medicine*, no. 98, p. 177, 1995.

59. V. Ng, "Serological diagnosis with recombinant peptides/proteins," *Clin. Chem.*, vol. 37, pp. 1667–1668, 1991.

60. M. R. Proffitt and B. Yen-Lieberman, "Laboratory diagnosis of human immunodeficiency virus infection," *Inf. DIs. Clin. North Am.*, vol. 7, p. 203, 1993.

61. J. M. Steckelberg and F. Cockerill, "Serologic testing for human immuno-deficiency virus antibodies," *Mayo Clin. Proc.*, vol. 63, p. 373, 1987.

62. A. Voevodin, "HIV screening in Russia," *Lancet*, vol. 339, p. 1548, 1992.

63. C. Farber, *Serious Advers Events: An uncensored history of AIDS*. Hoboken, NJ: Melville House Publishing, 2006.

64. T. Mossman and R. Coffman, "TH1 and TH2 cells: Different patterns of lymphokine secretion lead to different functional properties," *Annual Review of Immunology*, vol. 17, no. 3, pp. 145–173, 1989.

65. E. Maggi et al., "Ability of HIV to promote a Th1 to Th2 shift and to replicate preferentially in Th2 and Th0 cells," *Science*, vol. 265, no. 5169, pp. 244–248, 1994.

66. H. Kremer, "Did Dr. Gallo and his colleagues manipulate the 'AIDS test' to order?" *Continuum*, vol. Summer 1998, 1998.

67. J. C. Petricciani, I. D. Gust, P. A. Hoppe, and H. W. Krijnen, Eds., *AIDS: The Safety of Blood and Blood Products*. World Health Organization: Wiley Medical, 1987.

68. G. Schochetman and J. R. George, Eds., *AIDS Testing*. Springer-Verlag, 1994.

69. E. Papadopulos-Eleopulos, V. F. Turner, and J. M. Papadimitriou, "Is a positive Western Blot proof of HIV infection?" *Bio/Technology*, vol. 11, pp. 696–707, 1993.

70. V. Turner and A. McIntyre, "The yin and yang of HIV: A great future behind it," *Nexus*, Jan. 1999.

71. F. Barré-Sinoussi et al., "Isolation of a T-Lymphotropic Retrovirus from a patient at Risk for Acquired Immune Deficiency Syndrome (AIDS)," *Science*, vol. 220, pp. 868–71, 1983.

72. L. Stanislawsky, M. F, V. M. Neto, and et al., "Presence of actin in oncor-naviruses," *Biochem. Biophys. Res. Com.*, vol. 118, pp. 580–586, 1984.

73. D. S. Burke, "Laboratory Diagnosis of Human Immunodeficiency Virus Infection," *Clin. Lab. Med.*, no. 9, pp. 369–92., 1989.

74. D. Griffiths, "Endogenous retroviruses in the human genome sequence," *Genome Biology 2*, p. 1017.1-1017.5, 2001.

75. W. Vogetseder, A. Dumfahrt, P. Mayersbach, D. Schönitzer, and M. P. Dierich, "Antibodies in human sera recognizing a recombinant outer membrane protein encoded by the envelope gene of the human endogenous retrovirus K," *AIDS Res. Human Retroviruses*, vol. 9, no. 7, pp. 687–94, 1993.

76. J. Bruneau et al., "High rates of HIV infection among injection drug users participating in needle exchange programs in Montreal: Results of a cohort study," *American Journal of Epidemiology*, no. 146, pp. 994-1002., 1997.

77. R. H. Gray et al., "Probability of HIV-1 teansmission per coital act in monogamous, heterosexual, HIV-1 discordant couples in Rakai, Uganda," *Lancet*, vol. 357, pp. 1149–53, 2001.

78. S. Hugonnet et al., "Incidence of HIV infection in stable sexual partnerships: A retrospective cohort study of 1,802 couples in Mwanza Region, Tanzania," *Journal of Acquired Immune Deficiency Syndromes*, vol. 30, pp. 73–80.

79. N. S. Padian, S. C. Shiboski, S. O. Glass, and E. Vittinghoff, "Heterosexual transmission of human immunodeficiency virus (HIV) in Northern California: Results from a ten-year study," *American Journal of Epidemiology*, vol. 146, pp. 350–357, 1997.

80. C. Johnson, "Viral load and the PCR," *Continuum*, Nov. 2001.

81. K. Mullis, "Foreword to *Inventing the AIDS Virus*."

82. Z. Grossman, M. Meier-Schellersheim, W. Paul, and L. Picker, "Pathogenesis of HIV infection: What the virus spares is as important as what it destroys," *Nature Medicine*, vol. 12, pp. 289–95, 2006.

83. M. Irwin, "Problems with HIV Science." 2001. [Online]. Available: http://www.virusmyth.net/aids/data/miproblems.htm

84. P. Duesberg, "Retroviruses as carcinogens and pathogens: Expectations and Reality," *Cancer Research*, vol. 47, pp. 1199–1220, 1987.

85. P. Duesberg, "Human immunodeficiency virus and acquired immunodeficiencysyndrome: Correlation but not causation," *Proceedings of the National Academy of Science*, vol. 86, pp. 755–64, 1989.

86. D. Rasnick, "Noninfectious HIV is pathogenic." Mar. 1997.

87. E. Papadopulos-Eleopulos, "Geneva Presentation." 1998. [Online]. Available: http://www.theperthgroup.com/presentations

88. H. Bauer, "Demographic characteristics of HIV I: What is it about race?" *Journal of Scientific Exploration*, vol. 20, pp. 255–88, 2006.

89. A. Brink, *Debating AZT: Mbeki and the AIDS drug controversy*, Open Books., 2000.

90. J. Bergman, "Drugs, disease, denial." 2005. [Online]. Available: http://www.nypress.com/18/25/news&columns/bergman

91. C. Farber, "A daughter's death, a mother's survival." 2006. [Online]. Available: http://www.lacitybeat.com/article.php?id=3887&IssueNum=157

92. K. Mullis, *Dancing Naked in the Mind Field.* New York: Pantheon, 1998.

93. R. Scovill, "The Other Side of AIDS."

94. H. Caton, "The AIDS Mirage," Sydney: New South Wales University Press., 1995.